Healing Power

The True Mechanism of Mind and Illness

RYUHO OKAWA

HS Press

Copyright©2016 by Ryuho Okawa
English translation©Happy Science 2016
Original title: The Healing Power
All rights reserved
HS Press is an imprint of IRH Press Co., Ltd.
Tokyo
ISBN 13: 979-8-887370-48-4
First Edition (updated)

Contents

Preface 11

CHAPTER ONE

The Power of the Mind To Cure Illnesses

~ Lecture on
"Miraculous Ways to Conquer Cancer" ~

1. Each Person Has a "Report Book of Life"

   What determines whether or not an illness will be cured 14

   "Faith" and "space for practicing faith" are necessary to work a miracle 16

   Modifications to life plans can also be made 18

2. You Are Creating Your Own Illness

   God's domain that remains in medical science 21

   The human body is under the law of "impermanence of all things" 21

   What is the "astral body" that is designing the physical body? 23

3. What Is the Right Mindset to Cure Illnesses?

   Have a "heart of self-reflection" and the "feeling of gratitude" 26

   Put "the heart of loving," "the heart of repaying kindness" and "the heart of gratitude" into practice 28

Cure illnesses using your subconscious mind 30

  Tips to stop justifying yourself and choosing to be positive ... 33

4. Methods of Meditation that Repel All Illnesses............... 35

5. To Lead a Happy Life in Your Final Years
  A peaceful death that causes no trouble for your family 38

  Construct a future plan where you work actively with good health 39

CHAPTER TWO

Illness, Karma and Spiritual Disturbances

1. Illness and Death Are a Form of "Compassion" in a Life Plan

   The teachings of Buddhism are based on the fact that illness and death are unavoidable 42

   Death from illness is a form of compassion 44

   Worldly aspects also need to be improved to avoid falling ill ... 45

   Past life regression therapy is being used for sicknesses that cannot be cured by modern medicine 46

   Symptoms improve when the patients find the cause of their illness stems from their past life 48

2. Illnesses and Phobias Can Be Caused by Karma

   There are life scenarios related to past lives 50

   Atoning for past lives through the law of karma 51

    You will be placed in the same situation or in the reversed
    position as the past life 52

    The physical body transforms itself in accordance with the
    "suffering" within the soul 54

    Examples of influences from a previous life (1):
    People with distinctive birthmarks 55

    Examples of influences from a previous life (2):
    People with skin diseases, asthma or bronchitis 55

    Examples of influences from a previous life (3):
    People who are scared of water 56

    Examples of influences from a previous life (4):
    People who are afraid of heights 57

    Examples of influences from a previous life (5):
    People who are afraid of enclosed spaces 58

    Examples of influences from a previous life (6):
    People with panic disorders 59

    "Major karma," such as war, could also have an influence ... 60

3. The Influence of the Spirits Overlooked by Past Life Regressive Therapy

    In some ways, suffering in life serves to repay "debts" from
    past lives 61

    In past life regressive therapy, "past lives" and "possessing
    spirits" may well be confused 63

    Past life regressive therapy has insufficient understanding of
    spiritual aspects 64

4. Mental Illness Occurs Due to Possession by Evil Spirits

    You will develop the symptoms of the same illness as the
    spirit you are possessed by 66

Schizophrenia is a spiritual disturbance, not a disease of the brain ... 68

The electroconvulsive therapy at mental hospitals is a substitute for exorcism ... 69

Mental illness is a state where the physical body is occupied by other spirits ... 70

The spirits of family members or ancestors who are unable to return to Heaven cause spiritual disturbance ... 72

In the very worst spiritual disturbance, the patient can no longer distinguish between this world and the other ... 73

Demons and devils will repeatedly say, "I'll kill you," and incite the sufferer to commit suicide ... 75

5. How to Deal with Possession by Evil Spirits

Insufficient knowledge of the Truth and an egocentric way of life are the root causes of worldly delusions ... 77

The memorial service is more effective if you identify the lost spirit and pray for it ... 78

The difficulties involved in convincing a spirit and returning it to Heaven ... 79

It is nevertheless possible to cure serious illnesses and mental illnesses through effort ... 82

The effect of setbacks that are experienced at crucial moments in life ... 84

Consider an unfortunate illness or mental illness as a turning point in life ... 85

CHAPTER THREE
Q&A on Illness

1. Angina Pectoris was Healed by the Miracle of Faith ... 88
   - By experiencing an illness, one's view on life can change 89
   - The difference between those who "become ill" and those who "recover from illness" 91
   - If you have a goal in life, your intellect will not turn dull 93
   - There is no end to how much the human ability can be trained 95

2. People Around Me Have Developed Leukemia, Liposarcoma, and Uterine Cancer 97
   - Attain a minimal enlightenment about this world and the other 98
   - Regard the sickness as a challenge you have been given 99
   - Even when you are ill, make efforts to align your thoughts in a positive direction 100
   - Have faith in El Cantare and leave everything to Him 101
   - Create a vision of a bright future where your life changes for the better 102
   - Leukemia was cured by re-examining the work that did not suit the person's abilities and aptitudes 103
   - Atopic dermatitis was healed by finding the true cause of the illness 105
   - The virtue of *The True Words Spoken By Buddha*, which dispels negative spiritual influences 106

3. Nurses Should Use the Power of Words

Nurses have tremendous influence on their patients 108

Nurses should encourage patients with "words of light" ... 109

Medically speaking, I nearly died in my late forties 110

The unforgettable words from a nurse on night duty 112

My experience was reported as a "miracle" in a medical journal 114

The meaning of experiencing an illness 114

Cure illnesses with the power of the mind and the power of words 115

4. Miraculous Healing by *The True Words Spoken By Buddha*

Experience the phenomenon of evil spirits being dispelled, by using *The True Words Spoken By Buddha* 118

Drive out darkness by being exposed to Buddha's Truth every day 120

Tell people of various miraculous experiences 122

Have a heart to accept support from the gods and high spirits in the heavenly world 123

CHAPTER FOUR

Readings on Illnesses

1. Conducting a Reading on a Man with Atopic Dermatitis

A man who is suffering from atopic dermatitis for more than twenty years 127

The causes are the sense of responsibility and the wish for not becoming independent 131

Both the mother and son need to develop a carefree spirit 133

As a mother, accept that your son could be frivolous and
a bit of a "bad boy" 134

His own "workbook of life" comes prepared with important
points for healing his atopic dermatitis 137

2. A Reading on Alzheimer's Disease and Five Family Members with Cancer

Five relatives died from cancer and the mother suffers from
Alzheimer's disease 139

What the bereaved family should do to spirits that have not
returned to Heaven 140

Spiritual possession is the cause of Alzheimer's disease ... 142

The change that can be made to the fate of people
approaching the end of their life 144

Spiritual possession is involved if different generations
die in the same way 146

The virtue of a living person can save the souls to whom
he or she has some connection 147

Refine your virtue believing that you are "a life-saving
equipment with a rope" 148

3. A Past Life Reading of a Lady Who has Repeatedly Suffered from Cancer

A lady who was told that she was suspected to have breast
cancer after an operation for uterine cancer 150

A past life as a samurai with a strong sense of justice 152

She is reaping karma by undergoing operations 154

The virtue you must refine in this life is "tolerance" 155

The importance of shifting to a heart of compassion
and love 156

9

Afterword 159

My Illness Was Cured
By the Power of Faith! 162

About the Author 169
What Is El Cantare? 170
About Happy Science 172
Contact Information 176
About the Happiness Realization Party ... 178
Happy Science Academy
Junior and Senior High School 179
Happy Science University 180
About HS Press 182
Books by Ryuho Okawa 183

Preface

People's tendencies are mainly molded through the process of acquiring knowledge and experience. When these tendencies of the mind become fixed, they will create mental worries and sometime even go as far as to produce abnormal changes on the physical body. This becomes a "lesion" that sometimes manifests itself as incurable or rare diseases.

Modern medicine usually seeks out test results that vary from the norm, hypothesizes the cause of the illness and treats it accordingly. However, thinking about it, the illness is showing that our mind has strayed from the Middle Way or the Truth, which has resulted in certain deviations in our lifestyle and eating habits, or that we have continually been bearing heavy burden in work that is beyond our abilities. That is why, when conducting "life readings" at Happy Science, it often happens that illnesses immediately starts to collapse once its causes are identified.

The publication of this book may lead to a slight decrease in profits for hospitals, for which I apologize, but it will also reduce the government's welfare costs, and most importantly, when your illness is cured, you will feel the tremendous joy that cannot be replaced with money.

Ryuho Okawa
Founder and CEO of Happy Science Group
August 2, 2014

Chapter One

The Power of the Mind To Cure Illnesses

~ Lecture on "Miraculous Ways To Conquer Cancer" ~

Each Person Has A "Report Book of Life"

What determines whether or not An illness will be cured

This chapter is a lecture on my book, *Miraculous Ways to Conquer Cancer* [IRH Press]. For the past two or three years, Happy Science has been guiding our members to strengthen their faith, and as a result, we are starting to hear many people saying that their illness has been cured. Although I have assumed that the illness of our believers have been cured, after teaching about the causal relationship between "faith" and "recovery from illness," more and more people are being cured.

We have produced a booklet entitled, *I Have Been Healed!*, a collection of testimonials from our members who overcame illnesses through faith. As I read this booklet, I was surprised to know that even illnesses I had never heard of have been cured. But although it is surprising if you look at it individually, when you look at the overall picture, there is nothing really surprising about this.

There was also a special feature in March 2011 issue of our monthly magazine, *The Liberty* [IRH Press], about ways

The Power of the Mind to Cure Illnesses

to cure illness that even doctors do not know. Indeed, such cases are not rare.

Hospitals basically diagnose illness based on statistics. Doctors only observe various conditions such as gender and age based weight, height and so on as data, and look at various average statistical values. And they think that anything which deviates from those values is an aberration and therefore "bad," and start treating it.

On top of this, they also make various statistical predictions and are kind enough to tell us approximately when we are supposed to die. They calmly and hardheadedly tell people that they have a month, three months, half a year, or a year left to live, as if giving an "oracle" people should be grateful for. Doctors will give us "oracles," which would put fortune tellers out of work if they did the same. However, what the doctors tell us is actually a possibility based on statistics, and although it may be right statistically, it does not necessarily apply to individual cases.

Let me explain why it does not, using school examination as an example. In the case of examinations, some schools run mock exams and produce verdicts saying what percentage of a chance there is for each student to pass. Certainly, they can give an overall prospect of success, saying that there is an 80%, 50%, 20% or 5% chance of passing the exam, but the actual results of the exam will vary according to the individual.

Some students will pass the exam although they were given a 5% or 0% chance of success, while others may fail even if they were always considered to have an 80% chance of passing. There are also students who have always come top in exams at elementary school, all through first to sixth grade, but who fail on the last, crucial exam. These things do happen, when we look at matters on an individual level.

A similar thing can happen with illnesses. This is because there are actually factors that are not included in a person's individual data. For example, things like blood tests can measure physical data, but that information does not include what is inside the person's mind; in other words, their ideas and thoughts, or various spiritual influences. Thus, such things remain as unknown variables.

"Faith" and "space for practicing faith" Are necessary to work a miracle

In recent years, Happy Science has earnestly started healing people's illnesses. After all, to cure illnesses it is very important to establish our faith. If a person has strong faith, the healing of his or her illness will immensely speed up.

The healing of people's illness is also connected to the fact that more and more local temples of our own

The Power of the Mind to Cure Illnesses

have been built. If our local branch is located in a rented office amongst multi-tenant buildings, we can easily be affected by worldly matters, such as thought energies from businesses outside, making it difficult to create a complete sanctuary for practicing faith. For this reason, we need to construct our own buildings for a local branch, though we cannot ask too much.

Once we have our own building, we can create a perfect sanctuary to practice faith, making it easier for miracles to occur. It would be best if we could have proper precincts around the building, like traditional Shinto shrines and Buddhist temples, but since the price of land is rather high at the moment I cannot ask for that much.

Even so, at least it is vital to have our own buildings. In addition to this, it is also essential to establish faith in our teachings. These two elements will have an extremely strong influence on the effectiveness of healing illnesses.

In the Bible, when Jesus heals a sick, he asks the person, "Do you believe in me?" When the sick person replies, "Yes, Lord," Jesus responds, "According to your faith let it be to you," and the illness is cured. In other words, he is questioning a person's faith as the sole condition.

There are different levels in people's faith, and the outcome can change according to how high people have raised their level of faith.

Modifications to life plans can also be made

In addition to faith and the space for practicing it, of course the person's ways of thinking and the devotion to spiritual training will also influence the outcome. There is also a certain degree of effect from the spiritual discipline of his or her branch manager and ministers who offer prayers, as well as from the power of the spirits that support them.

Another influential factor is the intention of the spirit in the heavenly world who is responsible for our ritual prayers. There are many prayers and *kigans* (ritual prayers) at Happy Science, and all of them are guided by a specific guiding spirit. The effect of these prayers will also vary depending on how these guiding spirits perceive the situation.

In fact, every one of you have a "report book of life" of your own. This is something similar to "Facebook" that is very popular now. In 2010, a movie called *The Social Network* was released. It was about the creators of Facebook, a social networking service through which one can access to others' personal information, including names and faces. Apparently, approximately 600 million people around the world are using Facebook [as of the time of this lecture]. As a matter of fact, the "report book of life" that everyone has in the heavenly world is pretty much like this "Facebook."

I presume that Happy Science believers have experienced taking kigans at our local branch or shoja (temple). Suppose Mr. X from Local Branch Y, is attending the ritual ceremony for "Prayer for Eradicating Cancer Cells." At this moment in the heavenly world, the guiding spirit will say, "Mmm, Mr. X, let me see…" and, browsing through a book, will instantly find out information about the person's past, as well as what is scheduled next in the life plan he created before he was born into this world.

During this short moment of time, the guiding spirit will judge whether to leave the situation as scheduled, or whether to add revisions to the original life plan. When judging this, various elements such as the ones that I mentioned earlier, will be taken into consideration. Finally, a decision will be made as to whether to slightly alter that person's life, whether there will be no point in doing so, or whether it is after all worth doing.

However, even if the revision is made, sometimes the person would be offended to have his life on earth extended, since the other world is not a bad place. Upon returning to the other world, the person may get angry at the guiding spirit saying, "I was supposed to return to Heaven on schedule, why did you hold me back for ten years?! My final years were hard, and it would have been better if you had let me return early as scheduled." Therefore, making revisions to a person's life span will not necessarily lead to earning appreciation.

In this way, the guiding spirits in the heavenly world will instantly put together various information, and add their judgments in a moment's time.

You Are Creating Your Own Illness

God's domain that remains in medical science

An important thing I want you to be aware of is that fundamentally, you can create your own illnesses.

Today, there are many illnesses with its causes mostly unknown even in the medical field, and they do not even know why it appears. Modern medical science cannot even create a single Escherichia coli. They cannot create E. coli nor Helicobacter pylori. These bacteria appear without our knowing, and doctors do not know why. While they are researching on methods to kill them off by applying some form of treatment, they still do not understand why such bacteria appear. Various illnesses appear, and it is in this subject that God's domain still pertains.

The human body is under the law of "Impermanence of all things"

As I wrote in *Miraculous Ways to Conquer Cancer* (mentioned earlier) and other books, generally speaking, almost all parts of the human body are rebuilt within the course of a year or so; everything from the hair on your head to your skull, the internal organs to the tip of your nails. Apparently, many parts of the body do not even take a year, but change in about six months. This is probably quite hard to believe. It makes me want to ask how new ones replace the old bones. We certainly do not remove old bones and put new ones in.

Recently, progress is being made with new techniques to renovate and restructure buildings. For example, hotels are being partially renovated while still operating as a business, and schools are being partially renovated while classes are still being held. Normally a school would close down and classes would have to be held in a temporary building, but recent technical progress enables them to do partial rebuilding while classes are still being held in the school. In the same way, the human body completely replaces itself and all its functions within a year or so, while carrying on with its usual activities.

Thus, if an illness exists for more than a year, such as an internal organ having some kind of ailment, this means that the body is deliberately continuing to create that illness. In other words, it means that there is something there that corresponds to a blueprint to create that ailment, and spiritually speaking, there is indeed a blueprint that has this kind of function.

In any case, the human body is constantly changing, as stated by the Buddhist concept of "impermanence of all things." To use a metaphor, it is like the flow of a river;

although it may be the same river, the water that is flowing through it is most certainly not the same. Since it is constantly moving, it is never the same river twice. Please first recognize the fact that basically the physical body is also in a state of flux.

What is the "astral body" That is designing the physical body?

Each part of the body basically follows your own conception of what you are, and it tries to create what your thoughts are designing.

In some cases, even if the illness was not included in the original life plan, a design plan of an illness can intrude into a person's life plan during the course of life. This "design plan" is in fact the "astral body" that perfectly fits inside the physical body, and which leaves the body when the physical body is cremated after death. This astral body is almost exactly the same shape as the physical body, perfectly formed, right down to the fingernails.

The astral body is the outermost part of the spirit body, and an exact representation of the physical body, right down to each and every hairs and nails, and even to the nail parings. There is everything right down to the white crescent-shaped area at the base of the nails; it is possible to identify these tiny details.

The astral body is amazingly identical to the physical body, and its internal organs are also working. Even after death, its heart still moves, along with the other organs, with its lungs still breathing. This is because the person believes that he is still alive and, until the person truly understands that he is already dead, it continues to lead the same lifestyle as he did on earth.

In fact, this astral body forms the physical body, using various components such as protein and bones. Thus, when someone falls ill, the first lesion appears in his or her astral body. Something bad, that is to say, dark thoughts or ill parts first appear in the astral body, and then manifest in the physical body. This is the truth.

When such bad symptoms appear in your astral body, it is often the case that you constantly and repeatedly harbor destructive thoughts or self-punishing ways of thinking in your surface consciousness, or in other words, in your mind every day.

Or in other cases, you may have been very aggressive toward someone, getting angry or lashing out in discontent, but because that person's mind is pure, these aggressive thought waves are reflected back to you. If the other person is weak, he may fall sick, but sometimes he is not; when his mind is pure and shining with light, the negative thought waves that you emit toward him will simply bounce back and hit you. Thus, sometimes your own thought waves attacking other people bounce back and are hurting you.

This kind of spiritual cause does exist, and through clairvoyance, it can be seen that some kind of lesion first appears in the astral body. And it is after that it takes form in the physical body, causing lots of strange physical ailments to appear.

Medically, doctors will apply treatment from the outside, in other words, to the physical body, whereas religions apply treatment from the inside. That is to say, religions approach the issue by dealing with the original cause of the lesion, and begin by healing that part.

If you have become ill, that is most certainly because you have started to harbor some negative mindset in the recent years that do not stem from your essential true self. This is some kind of "attachment," and if you have some thought patterns that have solidified into a mental attachment, they will eventually manifest as a particular kind of lesion.

What Is the Right Mindset To Cure Illnesses?

Have a "heart of self-reflection" And the "feeling of gratitude"

When the waters of a river rise, the levee will burst and the waters will flow out. But the part of the levee that will burst is not always the same; it is usually the weakest point that breaks first. In the same way, we never know where the ailment will appear in our body. There are various kinds of illnesses, and it may be the heart, the kidneys, the lungs, the large intestine, the small intestine, or the blood vessels, that would be damaged. Just as the waters burst through the weak point in a levee where the resistance to the water is low or weak, so will illnesses emerge from the weakest parts of the body.

Therefore, you must start by changing your own self-awareness. If you believe that your body is like a body of a car, formed by combinations of external metal sheets and internal mechanisms, you will basically think that when it breaks down, the only way to fix it is to replace the malfunctioning part. However, your body is not like that at all.

The Power of the Mind to Cure Illnesses

As in the metaphor of a river, your body, which may seem like a car body, is actually changing every day; new materials are constantly poured in, and the old being eliminated. Thus, the body reconstructs itself as it functions.

If you have this awareness, you can recreate your body by giving your mind a firm direction in which to move forward. Of course, it is important that you give a good direction, not a bad one.

Nevertheless, in many cases people can hardly realize that their mental tendency is actually trying to create a certain type of bad mold. It is not an easy task to see ourselves objectively as if we are looking at ourselves in a mirror, and we cannot easily understand if our mind is distorted, or our ways of living is strayed. This is the reality. For this reason, it is essential to have the attitude of self-reflection and the feeling of gratitude.

Generally speaking, people who become ill have a surprisingly strong tendency to justify themselves, or a strong desire for self-preservation and self-defense. Despite having a strong tendency to defend themselves, they fall ill.

In fact, among those who become ill, there are many who try to protect themselves by putting a smoke screen around them, saying they are not to be blamed. Seen as a whole, there are also many who are offensive, criticizing other people and putting the blame on other things.

Such tendencies are quite common, so it is important to firstly have an attitude of self-reflection and the feeling of gratitude.

Put "the heart of loving,"
"The heart of repaying kindness"
And "the heart of gratitude" into practice

Once you have the attitude of self-reflection and the feeling of gratitude, rejoice in the fact that you have been allowed to live in this world. That is to say, rejoice that you were born into this 21st century, and are allowed to live up to the present day. Then, put your loving heart into practice toward other people. By actually expressing the love in your heart, your willingness to repay kindness, and your feeling of gratitude through actions, you will truly be able to change the "mold" in your mind. Therefore, it is important to put your heart of altruism into practice.

If you go to a hospital, you will see that most sick people are generally egocentric. It is very hard for them to think about anything but themselves. When you feel pain in your body and suffering, it is actually hard to think about others, even if you were told to do so.

Sick people are always saying, "It hurts here, there is pain here," and have lots of complaints toward their doctors, nurses, families, and so on. They also have various complaints and worldly attachments to their workplaces, or have various regrets about their work. No matter how good a person is, generally speaking, people become egotistical when they fall ill. This is usually how it is, and it is also an aspect of illness.

Therefore, if you do not want to fall ill, you need to construct a self-image that is opposite to becoming someone with an egocentric way of thinking. And if you find some mistake in you, be willing to practice self-reflection, and try to correct it little by little every day. You may find complaints and grumbles toward various people welling up from inside, but it is important to search your memories for things you should be grateful for, and to feel gratitude for any such things you find. Then, express your gratitude in words.

Furthermore, instead of centering your thoughts on yourself, think about what you can do to help people who are struggling, or ask yourself if you can listen to their worries. For example, if you have problems with your arm and the other person has problems with his leg, maybe you could help him by offering advice to him about his leg. In this way, it is important to understand other people's sufferings and sorrows, and try to ease them.

A little earlier, I mentioned the importance of having buildings for local branches; in a sense, the act of missionary work also means expanding the "sacred space" or "a place to practice faith." When the thought energy of many people gather and combine, it works to bend the rules of the three-dimensional world. The collective thought energies will twist and bend what is formed by the thoughts of individuals like a candy, and things will start to change. In this sense, to conduct missionary work and create fellow believers are also important.

Cure illnesses using your subconscious mind

In the final stage of illness, humans often become egotistical. In many cases, sick people end up becoming egotistical and pitiful, so please create in your mind an image of yourself that is the complete opposite of that, and be determined to be so.

Even if you do not get better immediately, it is important to believe that you are gradually changing in the right direction. By doing so, you are in fact planting an idea into your subconscious. Since you have to make it into a pattern, you need to plant that same way of thinking in your subconscious every day.

This works for matters other than illnesses as well. For example, many of you reading this may worry that you are unintelligent. Some may even keep telling themselves every day that they are stupid. Or, some may not be content enough with just telling themselves that, and say it to other people. I guess there are many who say that they are stupid, and do not feel satisfied until the other person nods in agreement. However, you will not get any cleverer by constantly telling yourself that you are stupid. Rather, unfortunately various phenomena will occur to confirm that you are not smart.

You may say, "Whatever I do is stupid," "I miss-saw the traffic lights. How stupid am I," "I didn't read the letter from the PTA asking us to come to the school for a meeting. How stupid," "I was going to have pork cutlets on rice for dinner this evening, but ended up buying curry and rice. How stupid of me." But if you keep reproaching yourself like that, you will not get any cleverer. It may partly mean that you are being honest, but it is not the way to make yourself happy.

Having said this, it would be a lie to say, "I suddenly turned into a genius today." So it is important to tell yourself, "I'm going to get cleverer, little by little, day by day." Then, once you find some change and improvement, praise yourself a bit. No one will become clever in a day.

The same is true for illnesses. If you constantly tell the aching parts of your body how bad it is, it will not get any better. Instead, you need to have a positive mindset where you say something like, "You've done your best so far. Thank you. We are going to be together for a few more years or decades. If you get better, even a little, I can do something for the world and repay my family a bit for all they have done for me. So please get better little by little, day by day." If you try doing this, your body will start reacting.

Internal organs are the typical examples of involuntary muscles. You may think that you cannot change them at your own will, and because most parts that become sick are involuntary muscles, you may believe that they are mostly uncontrollable. However, we can still have an influence over these parts that we believe cannot control. This is because, as I mentioned earlier, they are deeply affected by our subconscious. The subconscious is our mental tendency, so if we keep thinking about something for a long time, it seeps through the body.

I just spoke about how people worry about their unintelligence. If it was possible, they would want to correct the circuits of their brain through surgery, and make sure that there would be no problem with their brains. Some people may believe that this might be possible one day. They may expect that in the future they will be able to calculate swiftly and accurately by removing the stuff clogging up their circuits, or stow away everything they hear into a "storehouse" so that they never forget anything and can check it whenever necessary.

I am not sure if medical science will advance that far, but it is at least true that if you maintain your hope to be more intelligent, it will certainly come true. This is a characteristic of the subconscious. So if you want to improve your memory, for example, please continue believing that you have infinite storage shelves in your head. There may be times when you feel that there is too much to remember.

But keep imagining various information being stored in your mind neatly and in order, by telling yourself, for example, "This field is classified into this shelf, and that field is classified into that shelf." Then, you will eventually become able to organize and remember them properly.

Tips to stop justifying yourself And choosing to be positive

When doing this, you must be careful not to crush your hopes beforehand by complaining. People who have read our Happy Science books will probably understand what I mean. Human beings have the tendency to first have various negative thoughts. Although this is a painful fact and I do not really want to say this, humans are rather weak. We often try to justify ourselves, and want to find reasons so we do not need to work or do things for other people. However, this constitutes as a major cause of illnesses.

As I wrote in books such as *Miraculous Ways to Conquer Cancer* (mentioned earlier), when a company or a business goes into the red and goes bankrupt, for example, the president will often fall ill and even die. Of course this happens due to overwork, but it is also due to some kind of self-justification. In other words, he himself creates an illness to justify himself, in an effort to show that he did not fail due to his incompetence.

There are also people who become ill so that they can use it as an excuse, because they do not want to take responsibility for what is going on around them. There are even cases where people become ill in the space of one day.

Therefore, if you have the habit of making excuses, of justifying yourself, or running away from responsibilities, you must put an end to that. And you need to make an effort to engrave "positive thoughts" day by day, even if it is a little.

It is said that humans cannot think about two things at once. You cannot think of positive things and negative things simultaneously. For example, even if you were told to imagine simultaneously your car speeding along the highway at 60 miles per hour, and your car stuck on the highway with a flat tire, you cannot. You can only think of one thing at a time, and cannot think of both at the same time.

If you cannot think of two things at once, you have to choose one. So, it is essential to choose to picture a better vision or image in your mind, and to move toward that direction.

Methods of Meditation That Repel All Illnesses

Doctors will probably be astonished to hear this, but our internal organs also possess consciousness. For someone like me who has spiritual powers, it is possible to speak with the consciousness of the internal organs. When I ask internal organs where the problem is, sometimes they will give me a general idea of what is wrong. (See the aforementioned book, *Miraculous Ways to Conquer Cancer*.)

As human beings, our core consciousness center in the brain, but each part of the body also possesses consciousness. In fact, human beings are a complex composite unit, nurturing various things inside. Each single cell of their body is a living thing, and you yourself are "a galaxy." Human beings are like a galactic system, with many living organisms inhabiting a single body. This is something that you need to be aware of.

Please also know that your true nature is the spirit body. Gradually regard the physical body as less significant, and think strongly that the spirit body is the core and holds more importance. In addition, every night before you go to sleep, meditate on the spirit body as a golden orb, on your true self as a spirit body that is like a perfectly round golden orb. Your spirit body being "like a golden orb" means that it is perfect and flawless.

I would like you to maintain as much as possible, the image that your spirit body is essentially the precious life you have been given by God or Buddha, and that it is a perfect, flawless golden mass, a golden orb. By maintaining this image, you can repel any illnesses, from the top of your head to the soles of your feet. This "self-image as a golden orb" is your true nature as a spirit body.

When you die and return to the other world, you will retain a human form for the time being. However, when you ultimately attain enlightenment and ascend to the heavenly world, you will become a form of light energy shining in gold, like the golden orb. That is your true form. As you practice picturing your true form in this way, you will gradually develop resilience and resistance to various illnesses, or the ability to recover from them.

Flu, like influenza, starts going around in winter, and it is caused by tiny viruses. They do have a rather wicked face, but they are just tiny viruses. Those tiny viruses come trooping along; so the flu is a consequence of their "group possession."

A huge number of them come together. I do not know how many millions of them there are, but they come in masses like clouds, and penetrate into various parts of the body. So, influenza is a possession caused by malignant viruses. It is often said that you get better when you give it to someone else, and that is indeed true; you get better when they move on to someone else. The viruses will swiftly move on to a weak person. Therefore, as I just said, if you meditate every day on your self-image as a golden orb, these malignant viruses will go away from your body.

To Lead a Happy Life In Your Final Years

A peaceful death that causes no trouble For your family

In this chapter, I have spoken on illness in general, rather than focusing on cancer. Nevertheless, cancer is now the leading cause of death in Japan, and perhaps one out of three Japanese people are now dying from cancer.

Of course everyone has their life span, but I hope it becomes the norm for as many people as possible to lead a healthy life until their last day, chat pleasantly with their family, and then say, "Well, I guess it's time to go" and pass away.

Spending 10 or 20 years in hospital with lots of tubes inserted in your body, complaining about the pain and making trouble to your family, is very hard and is far from a heavenly situation. It is best to lead a healthy life until your last day, and go smoothly.

I have spoken about this before, but my paternal grandfather died a peaceful death of natural causes. At the time, my father's elder sister by two years, in other words my aunt, used to read him storybooks every night before he went to sleep. But on that night when she suggested that they continue with their book, he apparently said, "Not tonight, thank you." My aunt thought it was strange but decided not to read to him, and that was the night when my grandfather drew his last breath. It was indeed a peaceful death.

It is best to die like that, causing as little trouble for anyone as possible. That is what I hope everyone will experience. If you wish strongly, you can make your life move in that direction.

Construct a future plan where you work Actively with good health

The same holds true in setting the age for how long you want to work. Just like a work plan, if you create a plan on how long you want to work and start making preparations early, to a certain extent it is possible to make it happen. Sometimes it is not possible to prolong people's working life, if there is nothing for them to do when they reach that stage. Therefore, if you have strong feelings about how long and until what age you want to continue working actively, it is important to start making preparations at an early stage.

In my case, I am constantly receiving a lot of thought energies from many people, from all directions, wanting me to keep working actively for as long as possible and to keep on giving lectures right up to my last moments.

When people decide their work span without much thought, sometimes that will really be the end, so if you want to keep on working actively in good health, I advise you to establish a clear future plan for you to be able to do so. If you have nothing to do after your retirement, you may fall ill as a way to fill your time, so it is important to think of something that you can do.

A lot of what I have said here has been general remarks on illnesses. With these mindsets, cancer and any other illness can certainly be cured. This is the conclusion of my lecture on the book, *Miraculous Ways to Conquer Cancer*.

Chapter Two

Illness, Karma and Spiritual Disturbances

Illness and Death Are a Form of "Compassion" in a Life Plan

The teachings of Buddhism are based on the fact That illness and death are unavoidable

I previously had Happy Science branch managers submit reports telling me about questions from believers that they were unable to answer. Looking at those reports, I found that many of the questions the branch managers were unable to answer included matters related to illness and spiritual disturbances; particularly the difficulty in dealing with mental illnesses. So, I felt the need to give more lectures in relation to those matters. As one lecture is not enough to cover everything, I intend to talk on this theme in the future as well, and from various angles.

The first point I have to mention is that illness and death cannot be avoided. This is also a basic premise in the teachings of Buddhism, and is something we must accept. Even if an illness can be cured, it only serves to postpone death temporarily, or to reschedule the time of death. Ultimately, human beings die, and there is no escape from that. Some people may die of old age, but in most cases, people develop some kind of illness that leads to their death. We need to accept this as our destiny in life.

If we look at illness or death on its own, it may appear like a tragedy or a misery. However, from the broader perspective of the truths of life, including reincarnation, it is also a form of compassion. We need to be aware of this.

What would it be like if human beings had a sturdy physical body that never became ill? You can imagine the following case as an example. In the early 1900s, a black car called the Ford Model T was invented. The Ford Model T was the first car to be mass-produced in a standardized way, and it created the foundation for the Ford Motor Company to grow. However, what would it be like if those cars were still on the road a hundred years later? These are what we should consider.

Today, we have cars like Toyota hybrids on the road. Even if the Ford Model T were indestructible, would not get damaged even if people hit or kicked it, however sturdy it was, it would be natural for people to want to switch to a new car. As a matter of fact, people in general constantly switch to new cars. They want a car that answers their current needs, or the one that offers new kinds of performances. In this way, to be eternally indestructible is not necessarily the best choice.

Death from illness is a form of compassion

We humans want to switch to a new physical body when we undergo new soul training, just as we want to switch to a new car. We require a physical body that suits for a specific era, a new life plan and occupation.

To be able to make a new choice is, in fact, a form of happiness, and the price of that is the degeneration and death of the old body. Just as a new car becomes an old car and then be scrapped, the old body must degenerate and die. It is impossible for us to live for centuries in the same body, as if we are encased in something like a tortoise's shell.

Within the grand plan, dying from an illness is a form of compassion, and we need to accept that. This being so, it is essential to lead a fruitful and sufficiently happy life without causing people any trouble, like our family, or the people we are connected with through work. So it is only natural that we would wish to avoid collapsing with an illness at an important time, causing many people to suffer and creating new "hells" for our family. This is human instinct and is quite understandable.

Even if death is something that must be accepted, people would want to cure illnesses that are curable. If an illness is not curable, they have to accept it, but I believe religion can intervene to see if it has room for any chances to be healed. Medical science is probably aiming for the same thing. From here, I would like to explain the mechanism between illnesses and spiritual disturbances.

Worldly aspects also need to be improved To avoid falling ill

Happy Science teaches that about 70% of all illnesses are most likely caused by spiritual disturbances. But this depends on illnesses, and we cannot make sweeping generalizations. As the physical body belongs to this world, it can sometimes suffer "breakdowns" in a worldly sense.

For example, it could suffer from physical injuries or become incapacitated from playing sports. Anyone will certainly be injured if he or she falls from a high place, and those who have a badly balanced diet will damage their internal organs. If, on top of that, they do not do enough exercise, they will eventually get out of condition. People can become sick like this for worldly reasons, according to the general rules of this world.

There are also lifestyle diseases, such as developing diabetes as a result of consuming too much sugar. Nowadays, there is also metabolic syndrome. There are various indices for this, such as abdominal circumference of 90cm (35.4inches) or more for women, and 85cm (33.5inches) or more for men, high blood pressure, and other guidelines that need to be taken caution. Our lifestyles have become more affluent, but at the same time, these kinds of new illnesses have scientifically emerged.

To a certain extent, these symptoms can be observed in light of the rules of this world, and therefore it is possible to do something about them in a worldly way. If you consume too much food and beverage that are causing many people to suffer from illnesses, or if you lead a lifestyle that can make you ill, it is only natural that you will become more vulnerable to illnesses. You need to have this kind of worldly wisdom and improve what needs to be improved.

For example, people who consume excessive alcohol tend to fall ill, and heavy smokers are prone to illnesses, too. In this way, bad health has different causes. Worldly factors, too, can cause illnesses, so if you want to avoid becoming ill, you need to make improvement in worldly aspects as well.

Past life regression therapy is being used for Sicknesses that cannot be cured By modern medicine

Nonetheless, modern medicine is not omnipotent. Since doctors need to provide some kind of explanation to an ailment, they very often deal with illnesses by giving it some kind of name and telling the patient to take some medicine for the time being.

Medical science is still at a stage where more than 50% of it is "superstition." It seems to me that many of doctors' treatments involves providing a name to an improbable illness, or dosing the patient with medicine that does not work.

Looking at the patients' lives, some are suffering a sustained stubborn illness, or an illness that has a profound influence on their entire lives. In such cases, in particular, it is very common that the reasons behind these illnesses are not confined to worldly factors.

People create a life plan before they reincarnate into this world. Some may draw up an entire plan by themselves, but in most cases, they receive guidance from outside powers. In recent years, the Spirit World has also modernized, and in some areas, the spirits will watch their prospective life in a type of theater, as depicted in one of the Happy Science movies, *The Laws of Eternity* (released in 2006, produced and directed by Ryuho Okawa). There are also old-style areas in the Spirit World and things are somewhat different there.

In the U.S., there are psychiatrists that use past life regression therapy to heal illnesses that are incurable by ordinary modern medicine. As they apply hypnotic regression to a patient and allow his consciousness to return to his childhood, they find various things, such as emotional trauma that he suffered then, or parental violence and abuse which constituted to his current illness. And once the patient understands these causes, sometimes the illness improves remarkably.

Furthermore, there are cases where the patient traces back beyond his childhood through the hypnotic regression, and go far back as his time in the mother's womb and remember memories from his time inside, or sometimes even before that. This makes people think that past lives do seem to exist, and it has been a trend to use hypnotic regression to explore as far back as their past lives. However, apparently only a very small percentage of people are able to go that far.

Symptoms improve when the patients find The cause of their illness stems from their past life

Ever since this past life regression therapy started in countries like the U.S. and Canada, hypnotic therapy has been spreading fairly wide, and people are trying to seek the cause of their current illness within the stories of their past lives. This is one type of hypnotic treatment. Apparently, past lives are revealed rather specifically. They can specify which eras they previously lived, what their names were, and the kind of lives they led and how they died.

If we examine these cases extensively, we will find that in many cases, the causes of illnesses that cannot be explained with modern medical science are found in past lives. And it is reported that once these facts are known and the patient accepts and understands them, the symptoms rapidly improve and disappear. This is actually due to a kind of "dissolution of karma." The symptoms disappear when the patient becomes aware of why such symptoms appeared. As this has happened repeatedly, we can assume that such phenomena do exist.

This is a medical approach, and in religious terms, it corresponds to the practice of self-reflection. In other words, once you grasp the tendencies of your soul through meditation and self-reflection and reflect upon the causes of your illness, the symptom will start to improve.

So, it is becoming rather popular in the medical world to heal illnesses by using hypnotherapy in past life regressions, exploring its causes that lie in a patient's past life. Nevertheless, some source says that hypnosis only works for 4 to 10 % of the patients, making it ineffective for those who cannot be hypnotized.

Since the time of Freud, psychology has explained various mental illnesses as being due to factors such as abuse during childhood or infantile sexuality, but it is now becoming clear that the causes lie even further back than that. This is because many such cases have been discovered.

Illnesses and Phobias Can Be Caused by Karma

There are life scenarios related to past lives

According to past life regression therapy, there is a period called "interlife," or a life between the previous one and the next, and apparently, three "judges" often appear during this stage. According to an experiment carried out by a certain psychologist, they may appear in the guise of judges, old men, or various gods or angels, and in most cases, there are three judges. This is indeed very similar to modern-day trials. It is probably because there could be a bias if there were to be only one judge.

So, what happens is that three people appear and inspect the life you have just led in this world. They point out where the problems were, and help you understand these problems. And when you plan to be born next, they will advise you on the kind of life you should be living, judging by the previous one. Once you understand and accept it, you will incarnate based on that life's scenario.

This scenario includes an outline of your life in specific details, such as family relationships, occupation, whether you will die from an accident or an illness, and the age at which you will die. While it is truly mysterious, such scenarios do exist.

This being so, what you need to do is to look at your current situation in your life and think about the kind of life you led in a previous life that would possibly produce a scenario like the current one. This might emerge under hypnotic regression, but even if you cannot do that, you can find it through self-reflection, by contemplating on the possible causes for your particular illness.

Atoning for past lives through the law of karma

There are many experiences of the law of karma being confirmed in the religious field, and it also appears very distinctly in the medical field as well, through the above-mentioned approach. The law of Karma is usually apparent in the form of atoning for past lives.

For example, if someone abused or killed others through violence in a previous life, it is often the case that he or she will in turn be abused or killed in this life. In other words, if someone caused physical damage to others by the use of violence, like breaking and severing their arms or legs, there is an extremely strong possibility that he or she will suffer the same disability in this lifetime.

The same is true with family problems. There are many wives who suffer domestic violence from their husbands, but when such marital relations continue, sometimes the situation will reverse in the next life. In other words, the violent husband becomes the one that is abused, and the wife becomes the abuser.

The same goes for parent-child relationships. Sometimes a child who was abused by his or her parent is born as the parent in this life, and the parent is born as his or her child; so the tables are turned. There is also the issue of parent-child murders. If hypnotic regression is performed to a parent who murdered a child, or to a child who murdered a parent, it often becomes evident that the roles being reversed in a previous life. It is indeed terrifying, but the law of atonement emerges almost perfectly.

You will be placed in the same situation Or in the reversed position as the past life

There are two options for a scenario of the next life for these kinds of people; they will either be put in the opposite position from the previous time, or in exactly the same situation again to see what they would do this time. They will be tested to see what happens when the roles are reversed, or see if they end up doing the same thing when placed in exactly the same situation as before.

Suppose a man was brutal and violent toward women and was a rapist devil in a previous life. If he were to reincarnate in this lifetime, what kind of scenario would be created? If he had bullied many women and made them suffer, a scenario that first springs to mind would be to have him be reborn as a woman. So, one option is to have him incarnate as a woman this time and make him learn lessons on how he would feel when he is placed in the position of the victim. Another possibility is for him to be born again as a man in a position where he could abuse women, and to give him a chance to decide not to, through some life-changing event. Generally, there are these two patterns.

In particular, the experience of killing someone is engraved very deeply into the soul, so the person will be trained to see if he or she can desist from killing when placed in the same kind of situation once more. However, when it comes to the type of person who kills others no matter how many times he or she is tested, then a scenario that involves the experience of being killed could be included in the next life.

For this reason, although some events may seem tragic in terms of this world, there are cases where things have been planned to turn out that way. There are times when that kind of tragedy is necessary for the person's soul to learn lessons. In other words, sometimes tragedies occur as a result of what a person has done in a previous life that amounts to the tragic events in this life. If you think about this in terms of the law of compensation, you will be able to understand.

So there are two possibilities; being placed in exactly the same situation, or in the opposite situation. And those who make the same mistake again every time they are given a chance will be placed in the opposite situation.

The physical body transforms itself
In accordance with the "suffering" within the soul

Another element that often appears in the symptoms of illnesses in this life is how that person died in his or her previous life, which illness the person died from, or whether he or she died in an accident or by some other cause.

When some tragedy is engraved in a soul, the soul will be wounded and anguished by it for a long time. This anguish within the soul will seep out, even after it gains a new physical body in the next life. In many cases, this anguish alters the astral body, which then manifests as an ailment in the physical body.

Examples of influences from a previous life (1): People with distinctive birthmarks

In many cases, distinctive birthmarks correspond to the way in which the person died in a previous life. A great many cases have been reported where a birthmark appears in the place where the person had been stabbed with a sword, lanced or hit by an arrow in his or her previous life. The birthmark serves as a hint as to how that person died in the past.

Examples of influences from a previous life (2): People with skin diseases, asthma or bronchitis

The same is true with skin diseases. As the teachings of Happy Science already teaches, there are of course cases in which skin diseases appear as an allergic reaction in personal relationships, but if we explore past lives, there are also many cases where these are related to how that person died in their previous life.

For example, those who died in a fire retain a strong sensation of the whole body being burned during their final moments. When these kinds of people are reborn, they sometimes have a birthmark on their skin. It is also common for their skin to develop strong allergies in the form of various kinds of skin diseases.

On the other hand, people who died in fire and experienced extreme suffering, choking on the smoke are sometimes born in this lifetime with respiratory illnesses, such as asthma and bronchitis.

Apparently, when these people have past life therapy performed through hypnotic regression that I mentioned earlier, sometimes the ailments can be healed when they deeply understand that the way they died in a past life has caused their illness in this lifetime. This is truly incredible.

To put it another way, the mind is causing the symptoms that appear on the physical body. That is why when the mind, which is the cause, is corrected, the external ailment will be cured.

Sometimes the cause of asthma cannot be found in medical terms. But there are cases where it is cured when the patients understand that they have asthma in this life because in their past life they died in great suffering, enveloped with smoke.

Examples of influences from a previous life (3): People who are scared of water

There are also people who are very scared of water. They are scared of entering the water, be it a swimming pool or a river. They cannot help but feel fear when they see water.

If a life reading (spiritual research) is conducted on these people, in most cases they have died in the water in their previous life. It would be revealed that they experienced dying in water, either through sinking, a water accident, being killed with water, or dying in a flood.

If a person died like this, tremendous fear will remain in the soul. That fear will emerge as a type of phobia in this world. This is why these people are terribly scared of water.

Examples of influences from a previous life (4): People who are afraid of heights

A typical example is acrophobia. This refers to people who are afraid of heights. They become terribly scared when they go somewhere high up. When a "past life reading" is conducted, in most cases, they died by falling from somewhere high.

This could sometimes be due to war, or it might also have been from falling off a cliff, a roof or a scaffold; or falling out of a window, or of being pushed off somewhere high and killed. In any case, these people have experience falling from a high ground in their past lives, and they are hopelessly afraid of heights.

In the recent years, when those who died in an aviation accident are reborn, they will probably have fear with aircrafts. These people are terrified of getting on a plane, since the fearful experience in their past life will rekindle.

If they get caught up in a serious accident in this life once again, it will remain as karma. As the fear remains in the soul, this kind of phobia will tend to manifest in the next life when the soul reincarnates. Various things are carried over like this.

Examples of influences from a previous life (5): People who are afraid of enclosed spaces

There are also people who have claustrophobia. These people are scared of being shut or locked in. So they are scared to enter a small room or even an elevator due to terrible fear that they will suffocate. If a past life reading is conducted on these people, as you would expect, they have died in a way that involved being trapped and killed.

For example, those who were killed in the Nazi gas chamber will be very scared of being locked in an enclosed space. When there have been mass deaths like this, these people reincarnate fairly quickly. In many cases, however, they are born with this kind of phobia.

Or, if a spiritual research is conducted even further back in time, we sometimes find causes that even date back to Ancient Egypt. When a king died in Ancient Egypt, the manservant and the maids who served him were sometimes buried alive in his tomb along with the treasures. It was believed that the king would find life very hard in the next world if he was all alone, and that his retainers must follow him to the next world. So, they were buried alive and died in the pyramid, so that the king would be able to continue living as a king in the next world.

Without a doubt, they probably did not want to die yet, thus sometimes claustrophobia emerges as karma in their next life. Also, sometimes these people have a very strong fear toward being buried alive.

Examples of influences from a previous life (6): People with panic disorders

People who were killed in a surprise attack in their past life will suffer from things like panic disorders, and have extreme anxiety and fear. For example, they may have been ambushed by brigands while walking in the hills, killed by a mugger in a back alley, or by a burglar in their house.

I have just given several examples, and in a similar way if you find something that is unusual and cannot find any good reason for it from worldly causes, or if you simply cannot find any reason even in your childhood years, very often it is a manifestation of some abnormal experience that occurred in one of your past lives. Please be aware of this fact.

"Major karma," such as war, Could also have an influence

As I have explained, there is considerable importance to how a person dies. In this sense, matters like war create karma on a major scale, and therefore it is not very desirable. If you kill many people or a large number of people die because of war, this creates new karma, making later reincarnations very tough.

For example, if the development of nuclear weapons, by countries such as North Korea, leads to war and create a large number of deaths, we can assume that their next reincarnations could be a very tough life, because they carry over such karma.

When different ethnic groups kill one another, sometimes the ethnic group that did the most killing will, at some later date, be drawn into a war where a great many of their race will be killed. There may well be such reaping of karma on an ethnic level, causing such experiences to occur.

The Influence of the Spirits Overlooked by Past Life Regressive Therapy

In some ways, suffering in life serves To repay "debts" from past lives

If you suffer from an illness in which no reason can be found from a purely medical perspective, or if a particular illness has persisted for a long time in your life, it is often due to karma from a past life. Therefore, it would be a good idea to examine yourself, or seek advice from other people as to how they see you.

When a serious illness is involved, there is usually a life scenario behind it, and it is something that cannot be avoided. As I explained earlier, if you want to change that scenario, you need to think deeply about why this is happening, and resolve your own problems given in this lifetime. By constructing possible assumptions and trying to correct your life based on these, you may be able to alter the scenario.

Nevertheless, even if you cannot change your life scenario, in many cases, becoming ill and dying will serve as a form of atonement. It is something that had to be experienced, or otherwise you would have to carry that issue over into the next life.

For this reason, if you have treated people with extreme cruelty, committed atrocities, acted inhumanely or caused suffering in your previous life, your act of repaying your "debt" will be included in the pain you will experience in this lifetime. There are cases when your life issues contain these challenges.

However, although you may be suffering now, it is in fact something to be grateful of, because you are actually repaying your "debt." You are being told, "Your suffering may continue for years or decades, but that is because you did something that caused it in your past life. So, do your best to pay that debt in full, no matter how tough it is."

Sometimes poverty, illness, or conflicts in personal relationships, may cause you to suffer. Through this, however, you are actually "re-experimenting" due to your karma being carried over from a previous life, or you may be making atonements. Seen from a long-term perspective, the seeds of happiness for a greater span of life can be found in that suffering. Therefore, it is important that you try to perceive God's Will or Buddha's Will in your current suffering, and make sure to repay your "debts."

What is more, you need to accumulate "savings," and plant seeds of happiness for the future. It is not enough simply to repay your debts. You must lead a better life this time. Contrary to your previous life, you need to create "gains" and live in a way that will make other people happy. Lead a life that accumulates happiness this time. In this sense, it is important to be aware that you are being given a huge opportunity.

In past life regressive therapy, "past lives" and "Possessing spirits" may well be confused

In Western medicine, attempts are being made to cure various mental illnesses and disorders that are quite common today, using methods like past life readings and past life regressive therapy. However, there is something about such doctors that I cannot agree with.

When a person visits a psychiatrist with a serious illness, usually some form of spiritual disturbance is at work, and the patient is most likely possessed by a haunting spirit. For this reason, he or she should speak about this when hypnotic therapy is used. However, none of this appears in their report, but only the patient's past reincarnations.

I presume that the experiences of the haunting spirits possessing the patient are included in what the doctors believe as "past lives." While the stories of the ancient spirits may well be authentic, especially amongst the stories of those who claim to have been born in the past few decades, some may not be the patient's past lives. I cannot fully confirm this since I have not been present during a past life regressive therapy, but there probably is this kind of confusion.

To certify whether it really is the patient's past life, there needs to be a strong sense of the person's identity in the story. If that is not the case, it is highly likely that there is some spiritual disturbance. Doctors do not know much about spiritual possessions, so when they conduct past life regressive therapies, they cannot tell if a certain occurrence is from spiritual disturbance or if it is an actual event in the patient's past life.

Past life regressive therapy has insufficient Understanding of spiritual aspects

In past life regressive therapy, there is a short life called "interlife" between a previous life and the next one. It is said to be an extremely short phase, during which you drift aimlessly as if floating in the air, until you are born again.

However, the truth is that, as it is shown in the movie *The Laws of Eternity*, in most cases the spirits stay in the other world for quite a long time. Doctors probably do not really understand much about the life in the other world, because they do not have sufficient information about it.

What is more, it is also very strange that during past life regression therapies, Hell is not mentioned in the memories of previous lives that emerge. This is another point I cannot agree with.

There is absolutely no mention of Hell in the therapies. No matter the kind of life a person had led, he only speaks of how his soul immediately floats in the air after death, being greeted by a being of light, to reincarnate again not long after.

Seeing that there is no mention of Hell, no mention of the life in the Spirit World during the interlife, and no clear criteria to distinguish between possessing spirits and past lives, I presume that medical science extensively lacks information in these areas.

Mental Illness Occurs Due to Possession by Evil Spirits

You will develop the symptoms of the same illness As the spirit you are possessed by

In the previous section, I spoke about the insufficient points in past life regressive therapy. Religion adopts the position that spiritual disturbances do exist, and warns that living people can be possessed by a spirit of the dead. So, I believe that while an illness can sometimes arise as a result of a person's past life, it can also be caused by the spirit currently possessing the person.

If a person is possessed by a spirit that is unable to return to Heaven, the symptoms of the deceased person at the time of his or her death will appear clearly in the body of the person possessed. The person may suddenly develop an abnormally high fever, suffer an ague that makes him or her tremble violently, or develop other kinds of conditions on the body. The dead person becomes a haunting spirit, causing various physical symptoms to occur, such as cancer, a heart attack, asthma, or an agonizing headache.

I have actually experienced performing exorcism on such person; the moment I did, he returned to normal. One day, I received a phone call, telling me about a person who, while performing a memorial service for ancestors, suddenly started wheezing and gasping for air, developed high fever with intense cold sweats. I soon figured that a sprit has entered into that person, so I recited *The True Words Spoken By Buddha*[*] to the person from a long-distance over the telephone. The mere recitation of it made him recover, and he was soon able to walk around in perfect health. This experience made me assured that the symptoms of the deceased do actually appear.

A medical examination would classify this as a clear case of illness, but I actually experienced seeing how symptoms can appear purely as a result of being entered by a spirit that is unable to return to Heaven. After all, it is not the role of religion to utilize medication or surgical procedures; the religious approach is to heal any spiritual aspects of an illness that there may be. This is what we have to do.

---

[*] *The True Words Spoken By Buddha* is the basic sutra book of Happy Science. It is granted for those who became a member of Happy Science.

Schizophrenia is a spiritual disturbance, Not a disease of the brain

At the beginning of this chapter, I mentioned about the reports that I received from the Happy Science branch managers on their concerns. In them, I found a question along the lines of, "I have been doing my best to help those with serious diseases and mental illnesses, but I do not get any good results at all. What should I do?" This means that he is dealing with a difficult task, and he is facing a very strong opponent. Issues like mental illnesses, in particular, are perhaps the most challenging ones to tackle.

When a person develops what is known today as schizophrenia, his or her personality becomes split and dissociated. A child may start talking like an old person, or a man may suddenly start acting like a woman, or start using violence. The sufferer may sometimes rage violently or burst into tears.

There are also times when the sufferers try to commit suicide or harm their family members. Sometimes people around them are so terrified that they isolate them behind bars in mental hospitals. Such pitiful cases do happen. As there really is the danger that they might kill themselves, punch, kick, or knife others, there are certain worldly reasons in isolating them.

Doctors believe that this is a disease of the brain, but it is in fact caused by a spiritual disturbance, and unfortunately doctors cannot cure them.

The electroconvulsive therapy at mental hospitals Is a substitute for exorcism

The patients can sometimes be isolated and in serious cases, they can be the subject of electric shocks at mental hospitals as a part of therapy. This has practically the same effect as driving the spirit out or beating it out. In other words, when patients receive an electric shock, the spirit possessing them is also surprised and leaves them at once, curing the symptoms instantly. Thus, it is the same as exorcism in a way that it drives the spirit out of the patients. It is the same as what is called "purification" in religion.

There was a time when people flocked together and beat or kicked a person who had seemingly been possessed by the spirit of a raccoon dog or a fox. Sometimes it went too far that it killed the person. Such cases became a huge problem and were sometimes taken to court.

Actually, the electric shock treatment is practically the same as this act of beating out the spirit. Doctors are trying to treat their patients through electric shocks because they cannot perform exorcism or purification. They are actually giving electric shocks as a substitute of these acts, and it has practically the same effect. What is more, doctors prescribe the patients with medication that makes them lose control of their bodies, and try to stop them from acting violently. When the patients take medication, their body gets sedated and becomes unable to move. As a result, the symptoms no longer appear in the patients.

In this way, doctors try to weaken the patients' body through medication and administering electric shocks. However, the fundamental truth is that the symptoms are caused by a spiritual disturbance, which is of a serious level.

Mental illness is a state where the physical body Is occupied by other spirits

To use a metaphor, mental illnesses would be something like the following: Imagine there is a house. This house originally had windows, a roof, and a door, and there was a boundary with the outside world. One day, however, the front door broke and blew away, the windows smashed and the roof tore off as well. The original inhabitant still lives in the house, but because it is completely open to the outside world, robbers and burglars can now enter anytime.

This is the state of mental illnesses. There is no longer any barrier of protection, and anything from outside can freely get inside. The "walls" that used to protect the individual character are gone, allowing other spirits to enter the physical body anytime they want. Although the person's consciousness does return at some part of the day, usually other spirits occupy the body in turn.

The person's soul is connected to the body through a silver cord (a wire-like cord linking the physical body and the spirit body), so essentially it should be the strongest, but it oftentimes leaves the physical body. It would not have been a problem if it temporarily leaves the body while it sleeps, but because the person's soul ends up leaving during the daytime as well, the body becomes occupied by other spirits.

In severe cases, a person can be possessed by more than one spirit, mostly around five or so. There are also many who are possessed by around ten spirits. It is chaotic when possession is that intense, with the haunting spirits coming and going at their own discretion.

These spirits come to distract themselves in an effort to escape the agony of Hell. They come to possess the living because they want someone to listen to their grumbles and complaints. And they want a memorial service performed for them to find ease.

The spirits of family members or ancestors Who are unable to return to Heaven Cause spiritual disturbance

Sometime people say that mental illnesses are hereditary. However, they are actually not. There may certainly be people who are susceptible to spiritual matters, but spiritual possession is not something genetic. The truth is that, in the household, there is a flock of spirits of the family members and ancestors who cannot return to Heaven.

For example, an ancestor a few generations back may have died in a misery, and is unable to return to Heaven. In that case, the spirit will come to possess its descendants and cause some kind of disturbance, making them ill. Or, it might cause them to suffer an injury or an accident. Generally, in most cases, this happens to the most important or dearest person in the family, such as the child.

If strings of inexplicable accidents or injuries take place, even an average person would doubt that there is something wrong. Assuming that there must be some lost spirit, you may start holding memorial services devotedly for your ancestors. This is exactly what the possessing spirit is craving.

What is more, the possessed person will often end up leading an unhappy life and when he or she dies, this person's spirit will then possess the next generation of descendants. As a result, the number of spirits that are unable to return to Heaven will increase, from one generation to two or three, gathering around the family. They then possess the weakest person in the family, the one that everyone worries about the most, and say all sorts of things.

For example, sometimes a child abuses his or her parents, saying "Everything is your fault!" or "You made me like this!" If a child starts saying things like that, in most cases, the deceased grandfather or grandmother is the one who is speaking, or a more distant ancestor. Or, it can sometimes be the spirit of a parent's sibling. In fact, the possessing spirit is trying to put the blame on the people who are left, for the cause of its unhappiness. In this way, the personality of the deceased person takes over a living person.

In the very worst spiritual disturbance, The patient can no longer distinguish Between this world and the other

Even if the mentally ill person may appear to speak incoherently, what he or she is saying is in fact, "all true." It is just that the spirit inside the person changes. From the spirit's point of view, it is just expressing what it wants to say.

People with mental illness are actually experiencing Hell. Because they are witnessing the world of Hell while they are alive, they say things like, "Strange people come in here at night and talk to me." They do various things such as mutter to themselves or prowl around, but for them, it is actual reality.

The truth is that in the very worst state of spiritual disturbances, the sufferers are in the same state as a medium; they can actually hear voices of spirits, see, and sense them. They can no longer distinguish between this world and the other, and that is why they are sent to isolation. Those with severe spiritual disturbance are practically in the same state as a medium, but only strange and crazy spirits, not the high spirits, will visit them. Then eventually, their character will be taken over.

I think it is only natural that these people do not recover even if the Happy Science branch managers perform "Prayer for Exorcising Evil Spirits" or "Prayer for Recovery from Illnesses." That is because their "house" is devastated, with free entry from the outside. Their individuality has already collapsed, and it is extremely difficult to "rebuild" it.

Of course, there must have been some problems with the patients themselves, but their family members are probably not awakened to the Truth either. There is also karma from their ancestors that comes into play. That is why something immensely big has been manifesting. In short, the situation is that while many lost spirits are asking for help, the descendants do not have sufficient strength to offer help in any way.

Demons and devils will repeatedly say, "I'll kill you," and incite the sufferer to Commit suicide

Sometimes the patients are not simply possessed by four, five or six of such spirits. There are cases where, by visiting various religious groups, they end up "undertaking" spirits other than their ancestors; in the course of doing these rounds, they get entered by many lost religious spirits or other related spirits who are unable to return to Heaven, and thus things get more complicated.

Being possessed by the lost spirits of ancestors is not a severe case. Sometimes a person can be possessed by a demon or devil, which includes a malicious religious spirit. These spirits are sometimes referred to as "Death." When this kind of demon or devil comes to possess a person, it generally has the intention to kill him or her. Therefore, the possessed person will often hear the voice that threatens him or her to kill. The person will hear the voice saying things like, "I'm going to kill you" or "I'm going to kill your family," and that is exactly what the spirit is saying.

Eventually, the possessing spirit will actually make the person kill him or herself. When the person has committed suicide in this way, his or her soul is unable to return to Heaven and becomes a lost spirit, then goes on to possess someone else. Thus, a vicious cycle is created. Demons and devils keep threatening to kill or curse, so it is extremely hard to deal with them.

How to Deal with Possession By Evil Spirits

Insufficient knowledge of the Truth and An egocentric way of life are the root causes Of worldly delusions

The root causes of delusions in life are, "not knowing the right way to live, as in the teachings of Happy Science, during your time on earth as a human being," and "not knowing that the soul is the essence of a human, that the other world does exist, and that you become a spirit when you die." So, not being awakened to this knowledge of the Truth is the very cause of worldly delusions.

When they die, those who are not aware of these truths do not know as to what to do, as they still have life after death. They have no choice but to come to people such as their family. They have nowhere else to go, so they come to where they have a connection.

Another cause of worldly delusions is, "having led an egocentric way of life." In other words, the lost spirits did not live for the sake of others while they were alive. While Happy Science teaches the importance of giving love, those people did not put love into practice. They were egocentric and willful, did not give love to others, and thought, "There is nothing after death. Neither spirits nor the other world exist." These people take on the form of evil spirits after death and possess their descendants, causing trouble.

The way to deal with these spirits is to teach them the basic Truth in simple words, and the family members must also practice the Truth themselves. Furthermore, it is not enough for the family members to hold a memorial service on their own; it is important that they hold an official memorial service, guided by a minister, at a Happy Science local branch or temple. Happy Science memorial services will serve to correct the mistaken way of life and, at the same time, teach the truth of the Spirit World.

In addition, you also need to repeatedly explain to these spirits that they are piling up more evil by causing people to suffer out of their egocentric wish to be rescued, and that they must do good deeds instead.

The memorial service is more effective If you identify the lost spirit and pray for it

When holding memorial services, offer prayer to the individual spirits by providing their names, if possible. It is more effective in this way. Holding a memorial service for a vague target will not work, so if possible, it is better to hold a memorial service for an individual you know, such as your deceased grandfather, uncle, or aunt.

If an individual starts acting like a different person due to a mental illness, observe the person carefully and listen to what he or she is saying. Then you will at least be able to know if it is male or female. Then, observe his or her manners, since mannerisms that do not belong to that person will certainly emerge. Look at his or her hand movements, the tilt of the head, speech patterns, eye movements, conducts, favorite foods, and so on. If you find his or her gestures, way of speaking, and lifestyle closely resemble someone in your family who has died, that is probably who it is.

It is indeed more effective to hold the service for someone you have clearly identified. It is no good to talk in vague terms. As you observe their mannerisms, you may be able to guess, for example, "I know who it is. This is definitely my grandfather on my mother's side." Then, try and think about why he is deluded, and teach him the Truth.

The difficulties involved in convincing a spirit And returning it to Heaven

I also have some experience of preaching to the spirits that were unable to return to Heaven. They are in fact very stubborn, and it is impossible to correct their mistakes and convince them as a matter of mere 30 minutes. In many cases, it takes more than an hour. If there are five of them, it takes five hours; and if I do one a day, it takes five days.

Happy Science branch managers may perform "Prayer for Exorcising Evil Spirits" in a ceremony where there are 50 or 100 attendants at their local branch, but it is hard for it to be simultaneously effective on dozens of spirits. This is because usually they cannot return to Heaven at the first attempt. Even if they deal with just one spirit, it will take about an hour of persuasion to send it to Heaven.

To convince a spirit, you will need to point out its mistakes one by one, by saying things like: "You are the grandmother, right? You lived in a self-centered way; you were quite selfish, willful, and a miser who didn't offer any help for your children when they were suffering. You did nothing for them even when they were ill. You didn't help them, did you? In your later years, you constantly made selfish demands, grumbled and spoke ill of others. You caused a lot of trouble for others, and yet you didn't express any gratitude. Isn't that the way you lived?"

Correcting its mistakes like this would take at least an hour. You need to spend an hour or so to convince each spirit of its mistakes and send it to Heaven; this is usually how it is. If it is the spirit of a family member who had no connection at all with Buddha's Truth during his or her lifetime, it will not be able to understand even if it listens to the teachings of the standard level, or to the recitation of *The True Words Spoken By Buddha*.

Even though my lectures have strong spiritual power, if the spirits cannot understand the content, they simply would not want to listen; sometimes they try to flee or go in a rage. Videos of my lectures are the most effective, but when these are shown to the spirits, they would act violently. They dislike my lectures so much that they act wildly and start preventing their family from visiting a Happy Science local branch or *shoja*. Their resistance is extremely strong.

Therefore, when they cannot understand a difficult content, you will need to convince them using teachings of a more simple level. Since it takes about an hour to deal with one spirit, it takes an incredibly long time when there are five or ten of them.

If a branch manager were to take them on all by himself, he would be unable to do his regular duties at the local branch. It is this tough so I imagine the branch managers are using some simpler technics. A single attempt is not enough to help someone with mental illness to recover, or cure someone who has an illness caused by spiritual disturbance. Such issues are very difficult, so the family members must do their best as well. The whole process will actually take time.

It must be very hard to convince that types of grandfathers or grandmothers even if they were alive. Some people do not take others' advice easily, and that does not change after their death. It is therefore very hard to change a person's views on life and get him or her to reflect upon the thoughts and deeds of the past. It indeed takes a very long time.

It is nevertheless possible to cure serious illnesses And mental illnesses through effort

Even if haunting spirits are forcefully exorcised by dint of the Dharma power, they will come back again if they have not returned to Heaven. Unless the possessed person awakens to the Truth, he or she cannot do away with spiritual possession.

Once the spiritual possession has progressed as far as causing the person to suffer mental illness, the person's soul has become cowardly and scared, and is often detached from the physical body, even though its silver cord is still connected to the physical body. Therefore, the family members also need to help the person by praying that his or her soul and consciousness come back and take full control of the physical body. They need to send their thoughts, telling the soul to be stronger.

Tell the owner of the body, "Come back to your body and take control of it, for it is yours. You are connected to it by a silver cord, so this is your life. It is no one else's, so don't let others seize control of it." In this way, they need to help the person's soul understand this deeply and realize that it must take control of its own life. At the same time, they have to persuade the possessing spirits to leave, and detach them from the person.

Of course, when "Prayer for Exorcising Evil Spirits" is performed at a Happy Science local branch, the possessing spirits will temporarily leave, so it does have an effect. However, if dozens of spirits were present, simply performing the prayer once is not enough to ensure that they will never come back again. It even takes me about an hour to persuade one spirit to leave, and grandfathers or mothers from about a century ago will not be persuaded easily. Although it requires effort, you have to talk to each one at a level in which they can understand.

Therefore, it is essential for people living on earth to thoroughly study and practice the Truth, and undergo spiritual training. By doing so, they are moving toward the right direction, and so they could solve the issue. Through effort, even serious illness or mental illness can be cured.

This being said, however, in reality the issue is extremely severe, and in the process of tackling the problem, there may be counteractions; the sufferer may start acting violently, commit suicide, inflict violence toward his or her family members, or even go as far as stabbing them or setting fire. There are very difficult aspects to it unless you apply worldly wisdom as well.

There are cases where the sufferer is no longer him or herself at all, and in such cases, there may be no choice left but to put the person in a mental hospital. By doing so, the possessing spirit can no longer damage others and its power can be weakened. So, sometimes you may have to isolate the sufferer.

The effect of setbacks that are experienced At crucial moments in life

Having said this, I am afraid that doctors cannot truly cure them. Speaking in terms of the metaphor of a car I used earlier, this is the same as the car being so badly damaged that it no longer works. In other words, there are cases where an event in life has destroyed a person's personality so badly that there is no possibility of going back. I feel terribly sorry for such people, but there are cases like this.

People whose character has been taken over have most likely had setbacks in the important moments in their life. For example, they may have experienced setbacks in personal relationships during their adolescence, when they were at junior high or high school, or at university. Or perhaps their parents may have got divorced and the father or the mother left the family home. They may have lost a loved one through death; perhaps a parent or a sibling may have died.

Some people may have gone through a huge shock after failing an important exam, or have felt like killing themselves when love relationships did not work out, and fell into depression. They may have had to run away at night when their parent's business went bankrupt, or may have become seriously ill.

In other words, when you hate yourself or strongly deny yourself, your soul will want to move away from the physical body. Evil spirits will take this opportunity to possess you. Generally speaking, they can enter you at times when you hate yourself, hate your life, and hate the way you have become.

People become possessed at such times, when they have experienced a great shock in their life. There are also cases where they become possessed when they have involved with a strange religious group and a certain connection is formed.

Consider an unfortunate illness or mental illness As a turning point in life

Although these issues are truly complicated and difficult, the fundamental way to deal with them is to study the Truth and have the right views on life. It is essential to undergo spiritual training based on the right views on life.

Exorcism requires a certain amount of Dharma power,

so you need to call upon the help of those who have accumulated spiritual discipline. Please be aware of this as well.

Sometimes you may experience disastrous events in life. But try to minimize its effect and make sure that you do not carry over your karma into the next life. That is important.

When an unfortunate sickness or a mental illness occurs, it is actually trying to teach the family something. In fact, the possessing spirits are trying to tell their descendants that their way of life is mistaken. They are telling you, "If you continue that way, you will also end up like us." So, please understand such happenings in a positive way and take them as a turning point in your life. Make them an opportunity to correct your life, to reconsider your way of life.

If you do, poverty, illness, and conflict or strife in personal relationships will also serve as an entrance into the Truth, and a chance for you to find faith. They can be an opportunity to completely transform and rewrite your life scenario, as well as to pay off your karma from your past lives. I will be happy if you carefully consider these points and learn from this chapter, "Illness, Karma and Spiritual Disturbances."

Chapter Three

∽

Q&A on Illness

Angina Pectoris Was Healed By the Miracle of Faith

Q1:

First, I'd like to express my gratitude for the miracle that occurred through living a life of faith. To tell the truth, I was diagnosed with angina pectoris last year [2012] and went through catheter treatment. At that time, the doctor told me, "You were actually 99% on your journey to the other world, but you were saved because of a bypass vein that formed naturally on its own." So, I thank you so much.

RYUHO OKAWA:

Good. [*Audience applauds.*]

Q1:

After that, I decided to take various other tests to get myself checked further, and when I had my abdomen checked at a different hospital, they discovered that I had stenosis [contraction] in the celiac artery, which required an operation. But I was once again saved by the natural formation of a bypass. I am so grateful for you [*audience applauds*].

Up until then, I never paid attention to these things and just worked vigorously hard in high spirits. However, through this I realized that I could have actually gone back to the other world. So today, I really want to express my gratitude for this miracle. Thank you very much for giving me a new chapter in my life.

OKAWA:
No, not at all.

Q1:
When this happened, I strongly felt that we believers in "Living up to 100 Club" [a group in Happy Science that mainly consists of believers aged 55 and over] have a mission, and my dream is to spread this club worldwide. To achieve this dream, I am willing to study English with other members of the Club. So, I would be very grateful if you offer me some advice in realizing this dream.

By experiencing an illness, One's view on life can change

OKAWA:
It is perfectly natural that your illness has healed. It is not even considered a miracle here at Happy Science, so there is no need to thank me.

Nevertheless, there are good sides to illness as well. In some ways, you cannot understand how a sick person feels unless you have been ill yourself. By becoming ill, even once, you will become able to understand how it feels to be sick. You may become gentle and kind and your views on life may change as well.

Although I am essentially not the kind of person who should become ill, after I went through the experience of an illness on one occasion, I became able to do many "healings," and the number of people who have healed of their illness does not cease to increase. Until then, I didn't hear much about our believers having their sickness healed, but that may have been because I had never been ill myself and did not understand deeply enough how sick people felt.

However, after I experienced being sick once, I became able to heal people's illnesses very frequently. For example, there were cases where I healed someone's illness just by speaking to him personally. In other cases, someone's illness was healed just as I walked past him, without me even saying anything. Recently, by simply watching our movie, *The Mystical Laws* [released in 2012, produced and directed by Ryuho Okawa], people's illnesses have cured and gold dust sprinkled on them. In this way, various phenomena have been occurring according to people's wish [*audience laughs*].

I did not even expect it to have this much of an effect, but there are people who have been cured of cancer simply by watching our movie. This has not only happened in Japan, but in overseas as well, so this is not solely due to the power of words in Japanese. In this way, various sicknesses are healing all over the world. I believe that, as the power of everyone's faith grows stronger, this "market" will grow a lot larger.

In a sense, people who have had an experience like you [the questioner] can consider that they probably have a mission to work such miracles. In other words, they may have a mission to heal other people from their sicknesses. And people who have survived an earthquake can also consider that they probably have a mission to work such miracles for other people.

The difference between those who "become ill" And those who "recover from illness"

OKAWA:

Certainly, a bypass does sometimes form itself naturally. It is truly amazing that a bypass spontaneously forms when some other part become clogged.

After all, if one affirms an illness and wishes for it to become a reality at the depth of his mind, he will be drawn toward that direction. But if he doesn't want that, there is a higher possibility that he will move toward recovery.

Hospitals often tend to talk about the worst possible outcomes. This is because the actual outcome will not be worse than that, and people will be pleased when they get better. However, there are times when those doctor's words can stick to the patient's mind like a forecast of bad luck, and things can actually turn out that way. For this reason, people who don't listen to doctors actually seem to get better faster [*laughs*].

Doctors are very good at their studies and, like bureaucrats, they have a tendency to protect themselves. Thus, they are good at speaking in a way that absolves them of responsibility. This is why they talk about the worst possible outcomes. For this reason, while people who refuse to accept what doctors are saying generally won't die, docile and submissive people often end up dying. Therefore, if a doctor tells you that you only have a few months left to live, you can interpret that as meaning a few years or even decades.

Having said this, I'm not denying the use of hospitals. Happy Science might build one too, and I do not intend to express any opposition toward hospitals.

If you have a goal in life, Your intellect will not turn dull

OKAWA:

Regarding the mission of "Living up to 100 Club," if young people in the next generation work hard, bearing much responsibility beyond their age, there is a good chance that this activity could develop worldwide. It will be a very large project, but I do have high hopes.

You said that you want to start studying English, and I'm sure that you will do just fine. To tell the truth, I am becoming increasingly confident in my intellectual ability. I'm sure I will still be able to beat people in their teens or twenties in terms of intellect. The brain is a "device" that does not break down so easily.

The same is true for everything; if you leave something lying idle, it will only deteriorate. However, there will be no decline if you keep training it.

I brought along one of my books for today's lecture [*Shogai Gen'eki Jinsei* (Staying Active All Through Your Life) (Tokyo: IRH Press, 2012)]. When I read a book, I usually don't take notes. I haven't done so since I was around 30, and I still don't. I am actually able to memorize everything even if I don't take notes. I learn a book by heart simply by reading it. In this way, brainpower does not decline. It simply gets better, never worse.

Apparently, young people seem to have a hard time catching up with me, but in a way it is the role of us, the older ones, to train them. In this sense, I would rather want to say to them, "My, what bad memories you all have." [*Audience laughs.*]

At the moment I am producing a lot of textbooks on English words and idioms, and I heard that students at Happy Science Academy are being told to memorize them all by writing them out three times. That is the classic way to do it, and there is nothing particularly wrong with that. But I, myself can memorize everything simply by reading through them. I feel rather bad saying this, but I can memorize in a day what might take months for an ordinary person to do.

In fact, the end comes quite quickly for people who think that their work and studies are over when they retire, but people who believe that they get cleverer with age will remain fit. Looking at leading figures around the world, there are many who are aged 95 or so, and whose minds are still very sharp. This is probably because they have goals in life and have purpose in their studies.

Looking at my archives, I am now confident that I can continue writing books until I'm 100. It will be tough if I make it a duty, but last year [2012] alone, I produced 101 books that went on sale at bookstores. This means that I am accomplishing more work now than when I was young.

Two years before that [2010], I published 52 books and got into the Guinness Book of Records. Last year I increased my record to 101 books a year and broke the

Guinness record. I am actually concerned about what I am to do next. [In 2013, 106 books were published.] In any case, it is clear that the power of the brain does not decline if it is trained.

There is no end to How much the human ability can be trained

OKAWA:

The majority of our brain cells are actually asleep, and only the parts that have been trained gradually light up like lamps. Of course, these "lamps" do have durable life and some may die early, but there are still many other unused "lamps" inside your head. If you keep switching them on one by one, among the trillions of lamps inside your brain, you can continue to make them shine.

Therefore, if there is anything you were interested in when you were younger and think that you have still not gone deep enough into, or that you still haven't got a sense of accomplishment from it, it is never too late to start now.

Human beings have a surprising range of abilities. If we look around, there is so much talent being wasted in this world. You can definitely do better work from now on. Of course, a path will not open for those who make no effort, but you will become able to do things surprisingly well by praying for it and accumulating diligent efforts.

Particularly, when it comes to elderly people who have a great deal of work experience, it may be true to say that their stamina may have decreased a little, but in many cases they are superior to young people in terms of their work performance, or their ability to get work done. When these people tackle something new, they will become more able to master it in a surprisingly short time using their strong work performance. So, I hope that the members of the worldwide "Living up to 100 Club" will also make good use of this strong work performance.

Your memory will not at all deteriorate as long as you train it; rather, it will further improve through persistent discipline. So, you will not be outdone by young people for sure.

Please ignore phrases such as "Biologically and medically speaking..." or "Scientifically speaking...." Rather, it is better to tell yourself, "I am myself. I am myself and am directly connected to God's energy. I am now alive, directly drawing upon the energy of Buddha and God. By believing this, I can overcome any adversity."

I have high hopes for every one of you. [*Audience applauds.*]

N.B. The questioner's testimony of his angina improving after taking kigan (ritual prayer) is included at the end of this book.

People Around Me Have Developed Leukemia, Liposarcoma, And Uterine Cancer

Q2:

Three people close to me are suffering from severe cancer. One is my Dharma friend [a friend studying the Truth at Happy Science together] and suffers from acute leukemia, cancer of the blood.

The second is my brother-in-law, who is not a Happy Science member, but he has a rare disease called "malignant liposarcoma" which only strikes one person in a hundred thousand. The cancer is formed not in the internal organs, but in the fatty tissues around them.

OKAWA:

That means he is "trying really hard." It takes a considerable amount of effort to produce cancer in the fatty tissues.

Q2:

And the last is the wife of my colleague at work. Her uterine cancer has recurred. I really want to heal these three people.

You have been teaching us that the establishment of faith is very important to cure sicknesses, and that the patient's efforts also have an effect [see Chapter One]. What kind of mindset is required for me and other Dharma friends to concentrate the power of our faith and heal another person's illness?

Also, I have learned that by concentrating the power of our faith, the rules of the three-dimensional world will bend and no longer apply. How can we completely vanish the cancerous cells? I would be grateful if you could teach us about this mechanism.

Attain a minimal enlightenment About this world and the other

OKAWA:

If there are three people, their situations are probably different but anyway, they must first attain the minimal enlightenment about the relationship between this world and the other world. Otherwise, it is hard for the power of faith to work.

Minimal enlightenment means being aware that humans are beings that reincarnate between this world and the other. We currently dwell within a physical body and live in this world, but we are essentially beings that came from the other world and will return there. They need to believe that the spirit body is their true nature. I want people to have this way of thinking at the basis.

Regard the sickness as a challenge You have been given

OKAWA:

Secondly, in this world, many unpleasant situations arise in various aspects of life, such as human relationships, work or business, but they need to be aware that this world is a "school" and everything they experience will provide them with lessons to learn. This kind of attitude that I just mentioned, the view from the perspective of enlightenment, is necessary.

They mustn't be like a schoolchild who gets angry with his or her teacher for giving too much homework. Instead, they need to take on the challenge to find their own answers to the problem they have been given.

They need to accept their illness as a "koan"* and ask themselves why they have developed this illness, or where in this life the cause may be. If the cause is not in this life, it can sometimes date back to before this lifetime. It is important to think hard about the reasons behind their current condition, and to reflect on anything that comes to mind.

---

*Koan is a term used in Zen Buddhism. It is a question for contemplation to attain enlightenment.

Even when you are ill, make efforts to align Your thoughts in a positive direction

OKAWA:

There is one more advice. Although this is difficult for people who are ill, I want people with an illness to focus their thoughts on the act of altruism as much as possible. Even if they, themselves are currently ill, they can be of service to society, or do something for others, however little it may be. So, I advise them to make the effort to turn the "needle" in their mind to a positive direction, to a creative and productive direction.

If they focus on their illness, they will become unable to envision anything other than the image of declining and dying. By doing so, they will eventually end up trying hard to create a "movie" in which they are the tragic hero, or a heroine, causing tears to those around them.

Rather than that, I advise them to imagine a story in which they recover, give back to those around them, and transform themselves into a new person. I would like them to train themselves to elaborate this kind of image again and again in their own mind.

Have faith in El Cantare and Leave everything to Him

OKAWA:

I also advise them to study the teachings of Happy Science. The sick people may be in a state where they are unable to read books, but there are not just books but also CDs and DVDs of my lectures, so they can use these to study as well. By accepting and firmly believing in El Cantare, they will certainly come to understand that there is no sickness that cannot be cured.

After all, if people focus their mind merely on this world, everything becomes a source of anxiety for them and appears uncertain. But if they can firmly hold on to the El Cantare belief, they will eventually become able to leave everything to Him. Once they reach that state, they will probably find that their body suddenly feels at ease.

Although I have never heard of cancerous fat cells before, I have healed leukemia and have experience in healing most other sicknesses as well. So basically, there is nothing that cannot be healed.

Create a vision of a bright future
Where your life changes for the better

OKAWA:

In addition, in order to cure illnesses, there needs to be a reason to turn around the remaining years of a person's life for the better and to prolong it. Therefore, I advise people with an illness to think about building a positive future, and imagine the kind of future they want to create if their lives change for the better and are extended.

And I ask the people around them to support them in this. Sick people may often grumble and say negative things, but I would like you to think about how you can help them to turn that to a better direction.

Human beings have limitless potential. Even if the doctor says, "You are definitely going to die," it is correct to think, "I'm definitely *not* going to die." If the doctor says, "The chance of you dying is 80%," then you can think, "The chance of me *not* dying is 80%." If the doctor says, "The chance of you dying is 100%," you can think "The chance of me *not* dying is 100%." If you are told, "You have less than a year to live," then think, "I definitely have more than a year to live!"

Generally speaking, patients who deny what doctors say will live to an old age. This is clearly demonstrated by the statistics, and it is clear that people who don't listen to what their doctor says will live long.

The doctors see the sick and the dying day after day, so that is what they have come to expect as natural outcome. However, this is like a fishmonger saying, "Even if I stock up with fish, they just go off if they are left as they are." A good fishmonger does not focus his mind on the fish being left and going off, but imagines them being nicely cooked and bringing happiness to the people who eat them.

Thus, it is important to think about creating a bright vision for the future, and that is true for both the sick people themselves and the people around them. If the sick cannot come up with one, the Dharma friends around them could offer help for them to do so.

Leukemia was cured
By re-examining the work that did not suit
The person's abilities and aptitudes

OKAWA:

Our life span in this world may be limited, but we would want to attain a good state of mind before returning to the other world as much as we can. We wouldn't want to return by plunging down there [*audience laughs*].

We would want to die peacefully, at least knowing that

we are on the rise and at the right angle to enter Heaven if we continue that way. In many cases, illnesses make the mind negative and even drag those around the sick person into a negative mood as well. We must be very careful with this.

Cancer is the leading cause of death in Japan; it is a "national disease." It is the most common disease, so in a sense, anyone can create it for him or herself. But because anyone can create this disease, it is also a disease that anyone can heal. The easiest sickness to develop is actually the easiest sickness to cure.

I know a man who recovered from leukemia in about six months. He was someone who wasn't suited for management; he developed leukemia when he was assigned to a task that involved responsibility for a large organization. This made me think that his illness won't be cured unless he is exempt of that responsibility, and so I removed him from that position. Then indeed, his illness was cured.

Actually, it is very common for people to become sick when they are having a really tough time with a work that is beyond their abilities or a task for which they have no aptitude. This too, is something that needs to be considered.

Atopic dermatitis was healed
By finding the true cause of the illness

OKAWA:

Another important point is to exercise "divine power" to find out why an illness has occurred. For example, an illness that is caused by human relationships can be healed if the person identifies the cause and grasps the root issue.

I wrote about this in a book titled *The Moment of Truth* [Tokyo: IRH Press, 2014]. A while ago, in a Question-and-Answer session after a lecture at Hakone Shoja [one of the Happy Science facilities for seminars and spiritual training], I happened to be asked the following question: "I think I was an extraterrestrial in my past life. Am I right?"

So, I conducted a "space people reading,"* and I found that in the past that person had been a subterranean dweller on Mars, and hated going out to places with sunlight.

I didn't know at that time that he was troubled by atopic dermatitis that flared up with the touch of sunlight. However, his ailment was cured when he heard the outcome of my reading. His skin became smooth and was never bothered by atopic eczema again[†].

There are often cases like this, where an illness instantly "breaks down" when its cause is identified and understood. As the saying goes, "Onlookers see more of the game than

---

* Reading the soul's memory of an extraterrestrial who came to Earth to incarnate by using the six divine powers. See p.128.
† His testimony of atopic eczema being healed is included at the end of this book.

the players do," it's important for people around the sick person to tell them of anything that they suspect as the cause of his or her ailment.

Since you have asked me questions regarding three people at the same time, unfortunately I cannot provide guidance for each individual case. However, please don't bemoan that Happy Science has become too big to deal with each case in detail [*audience laughs*]. Instead, please consider it as lucky that you can heal so many people at once using our texts, such as the previously mentioned *Miraculous Ways to Conquer Cancer* [New York: IRH Press, 2015].

Every illness can be healed if I give individual guidance, and I used to do so at the very early stage of Happy Science. However, I soon became so busy that it didn't last a year. Nonetheless, as we now have a number of textbooks, we are starting to see many healings in various places by using them.

The virtue of The True Words Spoken By Buddha, *Which dispels negative spiritual influences*

OKAWA:

It is possible to cure most illnesses with spiritual causes by using *The True Words Spoken By Buddha*. They will be cured if you understand the content of this sutra book, and listen to its CD* every day. Even if you cannot recite it yourself, there is still benefit from listening to it. An illness caused by some spiritual influences will start to cure by constantly providing that input and removing these influences.

For example, it is very common for people to die from cancer if they are possessed by a spirit of someone who died from cancer. In such cases, the same symptoms that the person used to have will soon start to appear. This kind of thing can happen, so you need to help the sufferer understand the Truth taught at Happy Science until it reaches the depth of his or her mind.

In any case, the very fact that you were chosen to ask a question today means that light will now start to stream forth toward them. In my case, light will flow properly without me consciously "pouring" light onto a specific person. Your asking me this question today means that the spirit watching over you from "above" will follow you and take care of the people connected with you, so please make a proper request when you return home tonight. I'm sure that some form of change will start to occur.

---

* The recitation of *The True Words Spoken By Buddha* by Master Okawa is recorded in a CD. Not for sale. Only available to Happy Science devotees.

Nurses Should Use The Power of Words

Q3:

I used to work in the medical and welfare frontline as a nurse, but there was something that hit me, and I became a teacher at a nursing school this April. I intend to use my experiences to educate and train many future nurses. So, please teach me the ideal form of nursing in the coming age.

Nurses have tremendous influence on their patients

OKAWA:

All right. I believe quality is essential. Tasks and activities of a nurse can be copied and patterned, and so these can be taught to a certain extent by creating manuals. However, teaching mental and emotional attitude is not an easy matter. While it is possible to copy forms, since nursing deals with people, with many weak people in particular, each of the nurses' words or facial expressions has a huge influence on the patients.

Although the nurses may not think so themselves, for those who are seriously ill or on the verge of dying, they truly appear as "Angels of Light." The patients observe the nurses intently, trying to read the answers to their concern of "Am I going to die? Am I going to survive?" They stare at nurses, trying not to miss any words they say or any facial expressions and eye movements they have.

Therefore, people who are aspiring to become a nurse definitely need to do a deep study on the human mind. I am sure that it will be of use to them in their actual work.

Nurses should encourage patients with "Words of light"

OKAWA:

Happy Science certainly does not deny medical science, but the current situation is that the textbooks in Western medicine deal with illnesses only from a materialistic perspective, and do not even touch upon anything else. In other words, doctors do not understand aspects concerning the power of the mind. Surprisingly, however, nurses are not too materialistic and they are able to utilize the power of their minds.

Basically, doctors tend to start by explaining the worst possible scenario so that they will not have to take any responsibility. This tendency is similar to that of talented people. Those who are good at studies will tend to develop the habit of thinking about the worst-case scenario before anything else. As long as they are giving the worst-case scenario, when the outcome turned out to be better even slightly, they will be praised for their skills. That is why the doctors tend to give a dark picture.

On the other hand, nurses are not asked to take that much responsibility, so I would like them to encourage patients with Right Speech [right words], or offer them "words of light."

Medically speaking, I nearly died in my late forties

OKAWA:

I am now in excellent health, and quite amazingly, even a little stronger than I was in my early thirties. However, I once developed a heart ailment in my late forties, and medically speaking, nearly died. I had absolutely no intention of dying, but apparently, my doctor had "proudly" proclaimed that medically speaking I was soon going to die. I, myself was totally unaware of that and fully intended to leave the hospital very soon.

I had originally been hospitalized because they had found something "a little strange" in a physical examination. So I felt like I had been "trapped," since all

I had come for was a test. I hadn't had a hospital check-up for decades, and I sensed something a little unusual in my physical condition, so I thought I better have it checked once. However, when I went there I was hospitalized on the spot.

On top of this, I was told things like, "This is very serious" and "In fact, you are virtually dead already." My reaction was, "No way. How can someone who just walked in here on his own two feet believe that medically speaking he is dead?" In spite of this however, they attached a lot of cords all over my body and checked for various things, and I gradually started to feel they might be right and I started feeling anxious.

Doctors usually go for the worse options, so things were blown up out of all proportion and apparently, a rumor had it that I had collapsed from overwork. Moreover, it seemed like even doctors believed rumors and various rumors sprang up, such as that I had collapsed halfway up some stone stairs.

The truth was completely different; it was simply that my body felt a little heavy when I climbed some stone stairs during my walk that morning, and I just thought that I should pay a little visit to the hospital. However, apparently my family was told that with the state I was in, I might not see another day.

Meanwhile, I knew nothing of all that was happening. I asked my guardian spirit and was told that I would probably be discharged in a week or ten days. So I believed that, and casted away all worries.

The unforgettable words
From a nurse on night duty

OKAWA:

I still remember the words that a nurse on night duty said to me that evening. All she said was "I will never let you die." She was a beautiful nurse [*laughs*] [*audience laughs*]. She wasn't there the next time I went to the hospital, so she probably got married; but anyway, when that beautiful nurse simply told me, "I will never let you die," it made me feel very happy.

I had no intention to die either, but there was such a strange atmosphere around me. When I was eating dinner, everyone was staring at me as if I were a ghost. Apparently, everyone was thinking how impossible it was that someone who was on death's doorstep, medically speaking, should be sitting there eating his dinner with chopsticks in his hand. As I ate my meal, I said things like, "Is there something strange? This food is really good, isn't it?" because I had no idea at all that the doctor had said that I was dying, if not then, before the day was out.

The next morning, I woke up and got on with my work. I asked another nurse for writing materials, and wrote instructions to the General Headquarters from my sickroom. While I was doing that, the nurse who had come on duty that morning was looking at me in astonishment, as if to say, "He's still alive!" I had no idea why she was surprised and just thought that she must be mistaken about something.

When I do die, many spirits will certainly come to properly escort me back to the other world, so I will definitely know when I'm really dying. At that time, no such spirits had come, so I knew that I wasn't dying. A spirit in the other world had even told me the day I was scheduled to leave the hospital. So the next day, without any worry I started doing some physical exercise for rehabilitation, and apparently everyone around me was dumbfounded, saying that it was just not possible.

In the end, it turned out that I discharged myself to go home earlier than the regulations set by the Ministry of Health, Labor, and Welfare. I wanted to get out quickly since I thought I might be "killed" if I continued to stay there trapped.

Nevertheless, I was really happy to hear the nurse saying, "I will never let you die." I had gradually realized that everyone seemed to believe that I would soon die, so I was truly happy to be told like that. There may probably be people who really die, out of shock, when they are told that they are definitely going to die. Thus, words indeed have power.

My experience was reported As a "miracle" in a medical journal

OKAWA:

I am now in the latter half of my life, but it's rather "embarrassing" to have this much energy. It might be better if my energy levels were more suited to my years, but I just somehow seem to rejuvenate. It may be because the "energy from extraterrestrial beings" is infiltrating into me [*laughs*] [*audience laughs*].

I couldn't work this much when I was young. I would have collapsed if I had worked this hard then, but I'm in excellent condition now. In this way, many things that are medically impossible do actually happen.

This experience of mine was written in a medical journal as an "impossible miracle," using a pseudonym. Just like when any of you are featured in our magazine, I appeared under a pseudonym, with "age and occupation unknown." [*Audience laughs.*]

The meaning of experiencing an illness

OKAWA:

So, I was told by a doctor that, medically speaking, I am definitely "a corpse." I was then told, "You need to receive an organ transplant. At best, you will die within the year," and finally, "You have more than 80% chance of dying within the next five years." The doctors said all sorts of negative things, but all of them proved wrong.

The power of the mind is much stronger. To begin with, there was no way that I was going to die without my mission completed. It is absolutely impossible to die before my mission comes to an end. I now feel that I was probably made to experience illness so that I become able to cure illnesses; unless I experience it myself I would not be able to understand how it feels to be sick.

After that, I certainly became able to cure a lot of illnesses. People wouldn't be able to think much about the sick when they are in perfect health, so it may be a good thing to be slightly ill every now and then.

There are many religious leaders who have attained enlightenment after having suffered a serious illness and recovered. In this sense, it was probably necessary for me too, to experience an illness.

Cure illnesses with the power of the mind And the power of words

OKAWA:
I will say this once again: those words "I will never let you die" has firmly stayed in my memory. So words are truly important.

Healing Power

Sick people are all very anxious. They think about all sorts of bad things, wondering if their illness may be in fact even more serious than they are informed. So it is important to encourage them. Although telling them an obvious lie is going too far, it is essential to offer them encouragement. Humans are mental beings, so by harboring hope their illness can improve.

Incidentally, a doctor wrote something like, "Of all the hospitalized patients I encountered in my life, the one whom I thought behaved the most disgracefully was a religious leader" [*laughs*]. Apparently, someone who was said to be a high-ranked Zen priest behaved most disgracefully when he was carried into the ICU [intensive care unit]. He was thrashing around saying, "I don't want to die. I don't want to die." Be that as it may, religious leaders must basically train themselves to stand firm.

Anyhow, it would be best for the nurses to be determined to cure illnesses with the power of the mind and the power of words.

Doctors often give negative comments because they want to avoid taking responsibility, but that can sometimes worsen the illness. People like pharmacists also say things like, "You will have to take this medicine for the rest of your life." As it is their job to provide a constant stream of medication, it cannot be helped that they say things like that. However, human beings possess the ability to heal naturally. Most sicknesses are actually healed through natural healing, and not by medication. This is a subtle subject, which has a common ground with religion.

Thus, you will become able to heal illnesses if you are determined to cure them with the power of the mind and the power of words. Even if you are not a doctor you can sometimes heal an illness, because an invisible power will come to work for those who undergo spiritual training at Happy Science. Illnesses can be cured, so please bring the guiding spirits along with you as much as possible, and heal illnesses.

It would be wonderful if you could train nurses who are praised by people saying, "It's amazing how many illnesses can be cured in that nurse's vicinity." By training your mind, you can improve your ratio of healing illnesses by at least 25 to 30%. I have high hopes of you.

4

Miraculous Healing by
The True Words Spoken By Buddha

Q4:

Last year, you taught us about missionary work using "other-dimensional power"*. What should we do to exercise our true power, so that we can be of greater service to God and Buddha?

Experience the phenomenon of evil spirits Being dispelled, by using **The True Words Spoken By Buddha**

OKAWA:

Many people in Buddhist countries today are probably satisfied with traditional Buddhism. Even people who have faith might be thinking that they don't need anything else because there is traditional Buddhism. However, the question is whether or not people are actually saved by traditional Buddhism. For example, there are no reports regarding whether they are saved during their lifetime or after their death. This is the current situation.

---

* See Ryuho Okawa, *Ijigen Power Ni Mezameyo* [Awaken to Other-Dimensional Power] [Tokyo: Happy Science, 2012]

Traditional Buddhism has just become mere custom and habit, and people are simply saying, "This is the way it has always been done in our family." However, what is essential is the number of people who are actually saved through the traditional Buddhism. Happy Science is now providing accurate proof in regards to this point.

For example, a Japanese monk, Kukai [774 - 835], who founded the Shingon school of Buddhism, was able to freely use the mystical arts of esoteric Buddhism, and possessed strong Dharma power. Undoubtedly, he had Dharma power strong enough to repel evil and malicious spirits. However, his power was not passed down to his disciples properly. In that sense, it is doubtful that the Shingon school today has sufficient power to save people who are possessed by evil or malicious spirits.

Meanwhile, many people in Happy Science experience the repelling of possessing evil spirits and demons. They sometimes experience how the power of the Dharma manifests in reality.

Particularly, reciting *The True Words Spoken By Buddha* aloud is extremely effective, and there is also a CD in which my recitation is recorded. I actually use this CD myself as well, and although it's rather hard to say this since it sounds like I'm blowing my own trumpet and serving my own interests, it does possess tremendous power. Any evil spirits that are present will start to flee as soon as I get ready to play this CD.

It would be perfectly natural that they flee when the CD is played, but they try to escape as soon as I think of playing it on the CD player and start to make a move. So they must be terribly scared of it. The CD is about 20 minutes long and contains all the seven sutras, which are extremely frightening for the evil spirits.

At Happy Science some of my disciples possess psychic ability, by which I mean they can make spiritual phenomena occur. I play this CD whenever I feel the presence of evil spirits in them, and it truly does have an instant effect. They feel great pain and agony, and break out into cold sweat. Without a doubt, it probably feels like their entire body is inundated with countless bullets of light, or rather, arrows of light. This CD truly has tremendous power.

Drive out darkness by being exposed to Buddha's Truth every day

OKAWA:
The same is true with other books on Truth. Someone with spiritual sight once told me that my books piled up in bookstores appeared like a mass of light, and that is actually how they appear.

I started publishing books when I was still a member of the laity and worked for a company. I started with *Spiritual Messages from Nichiren*, and when I saw copies of my fifth book, *Spiritual messages from Socrates*, piled up in a large bookstore in Nagoya, where I was living at that time, I felt a flood of light pouring out from my books, and the air around them seemed to be vibrating. Even though they were only books, a flickering light filled the space around them. From this, we can see that books of Truth really have power.

Therefore, people who have *The True Words Spoken By Buddha* and other Happy Science publications at home, are protected to quite a large extent. At any rate, if you continue to make time every day to read my book, listen to a CD of my lecture, or watch its DVD, light will certainly pour into you.

In this world, unless you are careful, you will easily be tainted with negativity little by little. However, they will fall away once you start absorbing the opposite. Human beings are unable to think of two things at the same time, so if you can take in light, darkness will be chased out and fade away. It is important to continue this, and if there are an increasing number of people who experience this phenomenon for themselves, the number of people who understand Happy Science will gradually increase as well.

Tell people of various miraculous experiences

OKAWA:
Surprisingly enough, since Happy Science started out as an intellectual religion, in some ways, we have not spoken much about the miraculous phenomena, or proofs that bring believers worldly benefits, which other religious groups would announce right from the beginning. So, our publicity is rather weak.

We tend to think that publicity means running advertisements in newspapers, but religion does not actually spread that way; it spreads by word of mouth, from person to person. Therefore, it is important to tell people of various miraculous experiences.

For example, fist-sized cancers have actually vanished, and this is something that would knock doctors out for sure if they heard about it. They would doubtless want to say, "Don't be ridiculous. A fist-sized cancer has vanished? In just one day? That is ridiculous." But regardless of what the doctors might say, cancers actually do vanish.

In another case, a senior with senile dementia was healed by simply pledging devotion to the Three Treasures [vowing devotion to the Three Treasures of Buddha, Dharma and Sangha], and listening to my lecture on health. From the doctor's perspectives, such things are absolutely impossible. However, they actually do happen in reality.

Such miracles are regarded as perfectly normal in Happy Science. Our members have an inner serenity in a rather odd way, and accept such things in a relatively calm manner. People in other religious groups would go around talking about such things much more, but at Happy Science, it is perfectly natural and I even hear about such matters much later. Sometimes it is 10 or 20 years later that I hear about things which make me say, "What?! Did such things truly happen?" Happy Science believers are perhaps far too reserved.

Have a heart to accept support from the gods And high spirits in the heavenly world

OKAWA:

Even in cases such as the miracles of Lourdes in the South of France, the Church is very cautious about acknowledging the actual healing of illnesses. Although there are great many people who claim that a miracle has occurred, if you thoroughly investigate, only a handful of non-skeptical miracles remain, out of the huge number of cases that have been reported.

In other words, huge number of people go on pilgrimages to Lourdes every year, which adds up to millions or tens of millions of visitors over the years.

Apparently, however, the Church is conducting strict investigations, which only approves a few dozen within those people to have actually experienced a miracle. The Church authorities don't really want to acknowledge miracles since they are afraid of being criticized for being unable to actually cause such miracles themselves.

Meanwhile, various miracles are actually occurring at Happy Science. This is not simply due to the power of our lecturers or the head priests of our shojas [temples]. It is also due to the very power of the sutras including *The True Words Spoken By Buddha*, and to the current works and supports of the beings known as "gods" and "high spirits" in the heavenly world. This is where Happy Science's strengths lie.

It is important to know that high spirits are actually supporting us right here and right now, not just in some story of the past. Once you accept that fact, all sorts of phenomena will start to occur. Thus, in order to spread our teachings more widely, I believe that it is also essential to make many such happy phenomena take place in this world.

N.B. The testimony of a nine cm terminal-stage cancer being healed is included at the end of this book.

Chapter Four

Readings on Illnesses

"Reading" is one of the six divine powers, which are the unique qualities of someone who has attained a high level of enlightenment. There are various forms of reading, including "mind reading" where you access a soul's thought tape and read its consciousness, "remote clairvoyant reading" where you send a part of your spirit body to a particular location and observe the situation there, and "physical reading" where you see through a physical body like a CT scan, have a dialog with the internal organs and identify any lesions. Furthermore, in my case, I can clearly see things by specifying the time not only in the present, but also in the past and the future. This is a psychic power that transcends time and space, and is a blend of the ability of astral travel and the ability of spiritual sight, which are two of the six divine powers.

Conducting a Reading on a Man With Atopic Dermatitis

A man who is suffering from atopic dermatitis For more than twenty years

Q1:

I would like to ask you about my son's illness. He is now twenty-one and has been suffering from atopic dermatitis since he was two months old. Even today, the itching is terrible that it keeps him awake at night. We have tried various things we were advised were good, and even hospitalized him for treatment.

He also took *kigans* [ritual prayer], but there was very little improvement. He says that it is probably because his faith isn't strong enough. So, he has been reading your books and participated in Happy Science seminars. But his dermatitis seems to only have temporary improvements, and do not go away. Even the doctors couldn't find what the cause is when he was checked at the hospital.

RYUHO OKAWA:

No, you can't find the cause of atopic dermatitis at hospitals.

Q1:
Oh [*laughs*]. Also, since he was little, his symptoms seem to always worsen whenever he meets someone with the vibrations of evil spirits. We have tried various things but we still don't know the cause, so I'd be very grateful if you could offer us the direction we should follow for his treatment.

OKAWA:
OK, I understand. You said that your son is now twenty-one. What is his current situation in life?

Q1:
He's a junior in university.

OKAWA:
So he's a university student, and a boy. What is your family set-up?

Q1:
We are now a family of three. My husband has passed away, and the eldest of our three sons has already left home. It is my second son who is suffering from atopic dermatitis.

OKAWA:
So there are three brothers, and your husband has already died. When did he die?

Q1:
Fourteen years ago.

OKAWA:
Your son is twenty-one now, so if it happened fourteen years ago, he must have been around seven.

Q1:
Yes, it was when he was seven.

OKAWA:
What about the current situation of his brothers?

Q1:
My eldest son is now thirty-four.

OKAWA:
Oh, he is quite older, isn't he?

Q1:
Yes. He is already independent. My youngest son is eighteen and is a freshman in university. He also has a bit of dermatitis at times, but it isn't too bad and soon gets better.

OKAWA:
And you are the one who provides for the family?

Q1:
Yes, that's right.

OKAWA:
Just from what you have told me now, there is something about your husband that concerns me a little.

Q1:
I see.

OKAWA:
Did he die from an illness?

Q1:
He died of cancer.

OKAWA:
I see. Hmm. Although we are open to public, a reading would probably be the quickest way to answer your question.

Q1:
Yes please, if possible.

The causes are the sense of responsibility and The wish for not becoming independent

OKAWA:

Well, I'm afraid that I have to ask you for his name. His first name alone will be fine.

Q1:

His name is XXX.

OKAWA:

XXX. And he's a twenty-one year-old university student. Why does he have atopic dermatitis? Please give me some time. [*He faces his left hand toward the questioner, and holds just his right hand in the prayer position. About five seconds silence. He lowers his hands. About twenty seconds of silence.*]

Hmm... [*About five seconds of silence.*]

Hmm. This person is very "heavy." I mean he is mentally very heavy. This person is probably a very kind person by nature. I think he is a kind person. Although he is a kind person, he is just mentally very "heavy."

He takes many things to heart with mixed feelings, including a sense of responsibility for his father as well as his own, and for your future as well. He is a very kind person, and because of his kindness, he seems to shoulder responsibilities and excessive burdens. This is what I can feel from him.

I think that you should try not to worry too much about his dermatitis and his future. The more you worry and think about him, the more he wants to be a good son, and becomes even more pressured in finding a solution.

He feels very heavyhearted when he looks at his current state and considers how good of a son he can be to you and, as a working adult, achieve self-realization and be of service for the society. He feels these as a heavy burden, so it is better for you to help him feel a little more at ease.

Primarily, what is manifesting externally as atopic dermatitis will certainly decrease if you can help your son find ease. At the very least, he has a strong sense of responsibility toward what your late husband left undone. I can feel this burden he is bearing, so please advise him to take things easy. It would be best if you can remove his heavy burden by directing him toward becoming more relaxed and setting him free.

I can see that he has a tendency to agonize over many things he feels responsible for, so tell him, "It's all right for you to become more carefree and light-hearted. You don't need to think too seriously about all that matters. I'm going to lead a free and independent life too, so you don't need to worry about me."

One of the reasons he is suffering from dermatitis is due to his mindset that tries to prevent him from leaving home. In other words, it seems like there is a force preventing him from becoming independent from the family, trying to create extremely close family links so that he won't leave.

Q1:
Am I the one who is emitting those thoughts? Or is it my son?

OKAWA:
I get the impression that you are both resonating together. You are pulling each other.

Both the mother and son need to develop A carefree spirit

OKAWA:
Among people who study the Truth, some have a tendency to overly think of things in minute details, that they sometimes perceive things to be more serious than they actually are.

I suppose that your son is also studying the Truth, so one thing I would like to ask him is to make efforts to develop a slightly more carefree character. I would like both of you to become more breezy.

Unhappy events may occur in the course of life, but

there are many such cases happening around the world. A member from your family may die, parents and children may fall ill.

It just happened that in your son's case the ailment appeared as dermatitis, but it could have been other illness. It manifested itself in the form of dermatitis, which appears on the outermost part of the body. So this is actually not that serious. He could have contracted an illness that was more serious to his internal organs, but things didn't go that far and have not progressed beyond the external part. You should be grateful that it progressed no further than an external illness.

As a mother, accept that your son could be Frivolous and a bit of a "bad boy"

OKAWA:
The root cause here is most likely the sense of responsibility. While this is usually considered a good quality, his sense of strong responsibility is triggering his illness.

However, this quality itself is not bad, which is probably why it has not left him. In short, the strength of his sense of responsibility has become like a magnet, causing something on the surface of the skin to separate him from the outside world. This is the impression I get.

So what is it that you can do? Well, I don't really like to use this kind of word, but I would like you to become slightly more "frivolous." And I would like your son to be slightly more frivolous as well. There are lots of other people who have atopic dermatitis, so you should tell each other, "Let's be more laid back. Many things happen in life, so let's take things more easily. We don't want to end up with something worse after the dermatitis has gone, so let's not worry too much about it."

In most cases, atopic dermatitis is caused by human relationships, and sometimes it goes away once those worries are resolved. But I will refrain from touching on the subject of his relationships now. Nevertheless, I can at least say this: The fundamental cause lies in the way in which he feels responsibility. There is no doubt about that. This is the component at the core of the "magnet."

He really is a kind boy with a strong sense of responsibility; he is a very good boy. However, it is in fact because he is such a good boy that his illness won't heal. So please tell him that you don't mind him becoming a little more of a "bad boy." Please have some distance between the both of you so that he can feel he could sometimes be a "bad boy" to his mother's standing.

Young people normally do things that make their mother cry by the time they reach the age of twenty-one.

Being too good is not a good idea. Various "inconveniences" could arise in society when children are too well behaved, so tell him to occasionally do something that would upset his mother. Because he is repressing his feelings without doing such things, his dissatisfaction appears as atopic dermatitis. So, I think he needs to make an effort to live more cheerfully, and in a light-hearted way.

Yours may be a little different from a usual case. Problems in human relationship do also seem to be slightly involved, but I won't go into that because it might be a little embarrassing. In any case, his strong sense of responsibility and a gentle personality are at the heart of the cause. It seems to me that in a form of atopic dermatitis, he is trying to produce something in his appearance that blocks him from the outside world.

So you should rather think, "It's fine for him to be a bit more frivolous and a bit of a bad boy." There is no need to be praised so much by the people around you, and no reason for them to question your responsibility as a mother, so please become a little stronger. Take it more lightly to the extent to be able to say, "That's life, these things do happen. Dermatitis is better than cancer anyway."

The causes are around such matters.

His own "workbook of life"
Comes prepared with important points
For healing his atopic dermatitis

OKAWA:

Finally, we come to the question of whether his dermatitis is healable. In his life, there will be points where he will be able to cure it. One crucial point will probably emerge in issues with the opposite sex. On the next page of his "workbook of life," there will be issues with the opposite sex, and through his relationships, he will be facing hurdles to see if he can heal his dermatitis.

Therefore, although it may not resolve in this current point in time, I advise him to put effort to take things a bit more lightly. As for yourself, aim to become as bighearted as possible, without thinking too much on the details, and be accepting of what needs to be accepted.

I believe this case shows how an overly strong religious conscience can give rise to an illness. He is not a bad person, nor are you. Given that, you may think it is strange that he has become ill, but he seems to have things he must let go of. At the heart of it lies a sense of responsibility and, in a worldly term, a wish to make himself look better in the eyes of others. He needs to give these up as well. If he does, he will feel much more at ease.

Healing Power

As to whether his illness will be resolved, another hurdle will emerge when issues with the opposite sex come up next, and that will probably be a major turning point.

Having said this, ultimately, it is when he becomes ready to embrace his illness and thinks "It doesn't matter whether it is never healed," that it heals unexpectedly. It is often the case that an illness does not heal when people believe they can't be happy without a cure, but when people think they are happy even with their illness, it heals. So you need to change your ways of thinking a little, from one that is too clingy to one that is more free and relaxed.

I suspect that some cause also lies in the relationship with your husband, but I will not talk about that issue here because it is not appropriate for this theme. This time I have focused on your relationship with your son. Please try to live more lightly with a carefree spirit. This alone will surely make your and his lives much easier.

N.B. The son's testimony of his atopic dermatitis being healed is at the end of this book.

A Reading on Alzheimer's Disease and Five Family Members with Cancer

Five relatives died from cancer and The mother suffers from Alzheimer's disease

Q2:
This all happened before I encountered Master's teachings, but when I was still young, five close relatives including my uncle, aunt, and my grandparents died of cancer.

OKAWA:
Five family members!

Q2:
Yes. So I'd like to ask what kind of prayers we could offer for those who died of cancer.

And my mother is also slightly suffering from an illness that might possibly be influenced by that. She has actually been suffering from early-onset Alzheimer's disease from about fifteen years ago.

Also, I get the impression that many people who have lost a blood relative to cancer are convinced that they may have physically inherited a predisposition to cancer. So I would like to ask you how I should provide advice for such people.

OKAWA:
OK, I understand.

In old TV dramas and such, scenes that showed someone with cancer mostly led to death. In recent years, however, cancers are becoming increasingly curable so it does not necessarily mean death. Even so, treatment is costly and there is long-term pain, so cancer remains a symbol of tragedy.

Cancer is one of the illnesses that we can most easily contract. But we can also say that the easiest illness to develop is the easiest illness to cure as well.

What the bereaved family should do to spirits That have not returned to Heaven

OKAWA:
I don't think that there is enough time for them all, but if you can tell me the names of any of the deceased, I can examine where they are now within five seconds for each.

Q2:
Yes. First of all there is my mother's elder sister, A.

OKAWA:

Ms. A [*about five seconds of silence*].

Hmm, she hasn't returned to Heaven; but she is not deep down in Hell either. She isn't far down. She has not returned to Heaven but she is not far down in Hell either, so I think it is possible to guide her to Heaven.

Q2:

Is that so?

OKAWA:

She is within the range where you can save her by calling her name and teaching her the Truth in the course of your daily spiritual training.

Please tell me the name of the next person.

Q2:

A's elder sister, B.

OKAWA:

Ms. B [*about five seconds of silence*]. This one might be a little worse [*about five seconds of silence*].

I can see that she is still fighting an illness in a place like a hospital bed. So she probably hasn't been acquainted much with the Truth.

Q2:
She died when I was very young.

OKAWA:
I see. She believes that she is still sick, and it seems that she hasn't grasped her present situation; that she died of her illness and is now in the Spirit World.

I advise you to place an item or something connected with her nearby, such as her name written on a piece of paper, and send her your thoughts teaching the meaning of life, meaning of the soul, the significance of religion, what kind of place Heaven is, and the mental attitude required to go to Heaven. By doing that, it is possible to send her to Heaven.

Spiritual possession is the cause of Alzheimer's disease

OKAWA:
And the others?

Q2:
Yes. My relatives died when I was young so I can't really remember their names....

My mother is called C. She has been suffering from Alzheimer's disease for about 15 years.

OKAWA:

Alzheimer's for fifteen years [*about fifteen seconds of silence*].

She seems to be possessed by two spirits. There is one around her neck and another one on her head [*about five seconds of silence*]. They are probably not complete strangers, but spirits that have some connection with her.

Q2:

Yes. I did get the impression that it is someone blood-related.

OKAWA:

Yes, she seems to be possessed by two spirits.

To solve this issue, you need to perform ritual prayers such as the prayer to exorcise evil spirits or the prayer to send evil spirits to Heaven. It is such spirits that have come to her.

People tend to develop Alzheimer's disease when they are possessed; they often develop symptoms of dementia and the brain's chain of command goes out of order.

The change that can be made to the fate of People approaching the end of their life

OKAWA:
Is there anyone else?

Q2:
Yes. My father is called D. The doctor has said that he is fine, but he was told that the cancerous tumor marker values have increased slightly, and he is now taking medication.

OKAWA:
Roughly, how old is he?

Q2:
I think he's sixty-five now.

OKAWA:
[*About five seconds of silence.*] This person is within the range that can be healed. He is within curable range. He can still be healed.

Is there anyone else, are there any more?

Q2:
My husband's father is called E. He is eighty-one and he collapsed with a heart attack the other day. He suffered a

temporary cardiac arrest, but has managed to recover and is now at home.

OKAWA:

Eighty-one? [*About ten seconds of silence.*]

Hmm... It is quite "close." How much of recovery are people around him wishing for?

Q2:

Well, to be honest, given his age, we leave the timing up to the Heavens. However, if possible, we would like him not to suffer physical pain.

OKAWA:

Actually, he has entered the phase in his life plan where that kind of illness was scheduled. He has clearly entered that phase.

If there is some reason to change his fate, it is possible to add some slight amendment, but at this stage he has already entered the "target zone," so I could only extend his life by three to five years.

If the people around him have a good reason for his life to be extended and for him to recover, it is possible to modify his fate, but it would only be on a scale of three to five years.

Spiritual possession is involved
If different generations die in the same way

OKAWA:
Well, many things can happen in life and it can be hard.

Cancer is said to be hereditary, but I have to say that there are many aspects in which it just doesn't seem like that. Oftentimes all the members of a family with the history of cancer, die of cancer. Certainly, there are various things that are handed down in families and cultures, such as obesity as a physical characteristic or a liking for fatty foods in their diet. However, in cases where successive generations have died in the same way, it is largely not due to genetics but spiritual possession.

They die in the same way because they are possessed by the spirit of a deceased relative who is unable to return to Heaven. For this reason, I have certain doubts as to whether cancer is hereditary. In most cases, the spirit of someone who died of cancer is the one possessing.

In that case, you have to start by trying to remove that spirit. The whole thing is the result of the law of cause and effect, so you have to remove the affinity with such spirits so that they can no longer approach you. In other words, it is important to help the person cultivate and maintain a state of mind where he or she is on a different wavelength from such spirits.

The virtue of a living person can save the souls To whom he or she has some connection

OKAWA:

I feel that you, yourself, are currently on the right track. Your light seems to be fairly strong and since you emit a strong light, it may be your mission to save the souls of your entire family. I can sense such power. As you work hard to spread the Truth, your virtue will certainly be transmitted to them.

In Buddhism, it is said that when one person enters into priesthood, nine generations can ascend to Heaven. It means that when a family produces one person who becomes a monk, his virtue will affect around nine generations from their ancestors to their descendants. This is not only true for someone who joins priesthood; virtue that a person has accumulated by saving many people through religious activities will affect souls of those to whom he or she is connected. In other words, many will be saved in accordance with the virtue of an individual, and in the same way, people around you will be blessed with spiritual merit in proportion to your virtue.

For example, in this booklet entitled "I Have Been Healed!" [*as he picks it up*] you will find many testimonies of Happy Science believers on how their sickness has been cured, and to be perfectly honest, I don't know any of them personally. Since I don't know them personally, not one of them has come to thank me face to face, nor paid me a single penny [*audience laughs*]. Anyway, it is reported that they have been healed. My work is actually on a much greater scale than that, so there is no need to thank me each time something like this occurs.

Refine your virtue believing that you are "A life-saving equipment with a rope"

OKAWA:
I feel that you as an individual have a considerable amount of light, so if you continue accumulating virtue and sharing it with your family members, it will certainly serve to provide them with "buoyancy." Virtue is like a lifesaver ring against the forces trying to drag them down.

The reason why so many memorial services for ancestors are held is because a lifesaver ring flung by family members is easiest to rely on. After all, when a spirit is unable to return to Heaven, it first goes to its family members for help. However, if no one among its relatives possesses virtue, the soul would have no chance of being saved. If someone, even one person, emerges among the family who has refined virtue, it would be the same as a lifesaver ring with a rope being flung into the surface of the pitch-black sea, and the deceased would be able to take hold of it, trying not to sink, and climb it up.

The lost spirits will first come to their family members because those who don't really know about the truth of the Spirit World have no one other than family to ask for help. They cannot come to me, Ryuho Okawa, to ask for help. There have been cases where spirits trying to come to me have been repelled by space people in midair [*audience laughs*].

In any case, spirits often come to family members to begin with, so it is a great blessing if there is even one person who has virtue in their family. Therefore, while it is essential that you teach them the Truth, it is also important that you, yourself, increase your powers of salvation by accumulating even more virtue. This will enable you to save your family members, and you will also be able to save people other than your family members as well. So, please think of yourself as being like "life-saving equipment with a rope."

It is not enough to have virtue sufficient to bring happiness only to yourself. It is important to refine enough virtue to be able to save other people as well. I believe that you possess that much latent power, so please do your very best. Please break off the successive fate of cancer with your virtue. Please put an end to it.

A Past Life Reading of a Lady Who has Repeatedly Suffered from Cancer

A lady who was told that She was suspected to have breast cancer After an operation for uterine cancer

Q3:

I have been afflicted with cancer from about ten years ago. I developed uterine cancer last summer, and had my entire uterus removed. And recently, I have been suspected to have breast cancer.

I read your books and believe that I can cure my cancer on my own by correcting my mind, and I am trying as hard as I can. However, just as when I think that something good is going to happen, I always develop cancer.

How can I get the cancer to leave me?

OKAWA:

I see. If another cancer appears when one has been healed, that means it is metastasizing cancer, so it is like an endless chase unless you understand its cause.

Is it all right if I do a reading and investigate the cause?

Q3:
Yes, please.

OKAWA:
You can stay as you are. [*He puts his forefingers and thumbs together in front of his face, holding out his palms toward the questioner. About twenty-five seconds of silence.*] Hmm, I can certainly see something. [*About five seconds of silence.*]

I can do a "scanning" too. [*He lowers his left hand and hold out only his right palms toward the questioner. About twenty seconds of silence.*]

You seem to have a type of virtue.

So why does cancer appear and shift positions in this type of person? [*About twenty seconds of silence.*]

A figure of someone like a samurai is becoming visible to me. He is a samurai with a band around his head, wearing *hakama* [a man's formal divided skirt], and holding back its sleeves with a band of cloth. This is a duel, or if not maybe.... [*About ten seconds of silence.*]

Hmm, what is this? The opponent is not dressed in the same way. [*About ten seconds of silence.*]

This man has a very strong sense of justice. What I am seeing now is not you, but this samurai. A band of cloth is crossed over on his back, the cuffs of the *hakama* are tucked up and his sword is drawn.

He seems to have a very strong sense of justice. I can see him drawing his sword and cutting someone down.

The opponent is not a samurai. He is dressed like a townsman, but seems to be a gang member. I can see the samurai cutting him down. I wonder what the connection is between you and this samurai. [*About fifteen seconds of silence.*]

He seems to be driven by sense of justice and has made his own judgment, without taking any legal procedure. As an individual, he's carrying out this punishment on a seemingly villain man. [*About five seconds of silence.*]

There is probably money involved in this. The man he is cutting down what seems to be a moneylender and is collecting his debts. I can see the samurai cutting down the type who uses threat to collect his debts.

A past life as a samurai With a strong sense of justice

OKAWA:
This samurai is probably one aspect of your past lives. I can feel a very strong sense of justice coming from him.

Well? Don't you have a strong sense of justice?

Q3:
Me? Yes, I do.

OKAWA:

It's strong, isn't it? That is why he couldn't forgive that man and gave him punishment. I wonder what happened after that. I doubt that was the end of it. There is bound to be more.

Hmm. Ah, another opponent has appeared... It's just like watching a period drama.

Oh, I see. The cause of your cancer lies in the fact that you have cut down people with a samurai sword in your past life. That is the cause. The same number of cancers will appear as the number of people you cut down.

So, how many people did you cut down? Just now I saw you cut down the first one, the townsman. Now I can see the second one, who doesn't look like a townsman, coming onto the scene. He looks to be a guard man. I suppose the boss of the moneylenders is somewhere in the background.

At this stage, I don't know just how far you went, but the same number of cancers will probably develop as the number of people you cut down. But I don't think there were that many of them, and it might have been only two [*he lowers the hand held against the questioner*].

She is reaping karma by undergoing operations

OKAWA:
It is common for people who caused bloodshed with a blade in a past life to develop illnesses that require surgery. This does not necessarily have any relation to whether they are a good person or a bad person. It does not mean that because you are a good person, you don't get sick, or because you're a bad person, you get sick.

There have been many eras of warfare in the past, and depending on the era in which they are born, people were sometimes drawn into bloodshed whether they like it or not. In such cases, it is common for them to suffer from an illness that requires surgery. This scenario of "being cut" can be included in their "workbook of life." My father, too, had more or less this aspect.

Thus, the cause of your cancer is that you have cut down people with a samurai sword in a past life. However, you were not a villain. You had a burning sense of justice, and you acted for a good cause. There was probably some kind of injustice, which was not corrected, and so you were driven by righteousness to give out punishment yourself.

In today's reading, I could see that you had got as far as punishing a second person, but the boss would still be there behind the scene and I don't know how far you ultimately got. Still, I don't think it would have been more than two. That's probably about it.

The virtue you must refine in this life Is "tolerance"

OKAWA:

Just now, I did a past life reading [illness reading] to explore the reason why you have cancer. This is also called "karma reading." In short, if a person injured others with a blade, he will most likely create karma that leads him to have surgery in a next life, and that is the cause in your case as well.

You have a very strong sense of justice, and I think that you are fundamentally a good person. However, your hatred toward evil is so extreme that you want to pin down what is evil, even harsher than an average man. I believe you display that soul's tendency in this lifetime as well.

Nevertheless, you cannot take responsibility in this lifetime for what you did in the past life. Swords are no longer used in the modern era, so you can't do anything with it. Therefore, what you should do now is this: If you are "cutting people down" with your words instead of a sword, you need to observe the teachings of Right Speech more closely and better your language.

And, rather than just erasing the negative trait, it is also important to develop a new positive one. People with a strong sense of justice need to refine the virtue of "tolerance," as an opposite trait, and it is important for them to increase their capacity to accept other people.

From now on, please try to boost your tolerance even more, and pay attention to Right Speech, in other words, bettering your language. You probably want to clearly classify people into "good" and "bad," but in each person there are sides that other people cannot see. So, from now on, make effort to be able to see these hidden sides in people. Doing so will surely enhance your virtue.

These things I have just told you are what you need to do now. So you don't need to do anything about the event that occurred in your past life.

The importance of shifting to a heart of Compassion and love

OKAWA:
Before people reincarnate into this world, they often write and include "reaping of karma" into their life plan. If they think, "In my opinion, I would like to eliminate this area of guilt during this lifetime," sometimes they include hardships such as illness in their life plan.

In this reading, I could clearly see a samurai cutting someone down. That must be the cause of your cancer, but that has nothing to do with you directly in this lifetime.

So what you can do now is to further elevate your state of mind, soften your mind, and nurture a heart of tolerance. Although it is good to have a strong sense of justice, it is important that from now on you make a slight shift in the direction of developing a heart of love and a heart of compassion. These efforts will certainly put a stop to your cancer.

N.B. Her testimony of the metastasis of her cancer, that stopped after the reading, is included at the end of this book.

Afterword

Today, people tend to believe that illnesses can be cured by doctor's treatment and medication, so it is no doubt that they are amazed to know that my words alone can make fist-sized cancers disappear, and that incurable diseases are healed by me simply walking past the sick at a Happy Science local branch. I also keep hearing stories such as an elderly person who had to use crutches for many years threw them away and walked home briskly when I made a visit to their newly built local temple. There are even people whose illness has been cured simply by watching a Happy Science movie.

I am a rational man who received a modern-day education. There is absolutely no cheating or trickery involved. The people themselves and those around them see it as "a miracle" because they do not yet know the power of faith. If Jesus, the founder of Christianity, could do so much healing, just imagine what his spiritual father, El Cantare, is capable of.

The guiding principles in this book can also be useful for doctors and nurses, and they can of course use them at hospitals.

Ryuho Okawa
Founder and CEO of Happy Science Group
August 2, 2014

This book is a compilation of the lectures and
Q&A sessions, with additions, as listed below.

- CHAPTER ONE -
The Power of the Mind to Cure Illnesses
~ Lecture on "Miraculous Ways to Conquer Cancer" ~

Lecture given on February 6, 2011
at Yokohama Totsuka Local Temple, Kanagawa, Japan

- CHAPTER TWO -
Illness, Karma and Spiritual Disturbances

Lecture given on October 24, 2006
at Happy Science General Headquarters, Tokyo, Japan

- CHAPTER THREE -
Q&A on Illness

1. Angina Pectoris was Healed by the Miracle of Faith

Q&A conducted on January 27, 2013
at Head Temple Shoshinkan, Tochigi, Japan

2. People Around Me Have Developed Leukemia, Liposarcoma, and Uterine Cancer

Q&A conducted on February 6, 2011
at Yokohama Totsuka Local Temple, Kanagawa, Japan

3. Nurses Should Use the Power of Words

Q&A conducted on April 10, 2011
at Okayama Higashi Local Temple, Okayama, Japan

4. Miraculous Healing by *The True Words Spoken By Buddha*

Q&A conducted on February 21, 2010
at Naruto Local Temple, Tokushima, Japan

- CHAPTER FOUR -
Readings on Illnesses

1. Conducting a Reading on a Man with Atopic Dermatitis

Q&A conducted on October 23, 2011
at Tokyo Shoshinkan, Tokyo, Japan

2. A Reading on Alzheimer's Disease and Five Family Members with Cancer

Q&A conducted on February 6, 2011
at Yokohama Totsuka Local Temple, Kanagawa, Japan

3. A Past Life Reading of a Lady Who has Repeatedly Suffered from Cancer

Same as above

My Illness Was Cured by the Power of Faith!

People are experiencing miracles one after another

At Happy Science, there have been various reports from worldwide of people's illnesses miraculously curing. We would like to introduce some of the testimonies given by these people who overcame their life's problems by using the power of faith.

Testimony 1
Following up on the questioner from Ch. 4.

BY CHANGING OUR MINDS, MY SECOND SON'S ATOPIC DERMATITIS WAS HEALED!

"My second son started to have atopic dermatitis when he was two months old. His distressing symptoms continued even after he became a university student. So I summoned my courage and asked Master Okawa about this problem, and he conducted a reading on our personality and our life plan, providing us with advice on how we should think. We made an effort to change our thoughts exactly as Master Ryuho Okawa had said, and my son's atopic dermatitis started to heal dramatically. Currently, he is almost fully healed, to a point where his skin has a glow. I am grateful from the bottom of my heart."

(Ms. M.T.)

Testimony 2 — MY METASTASIZING CANCER STOPPED AFTER MY PAST LIFE READING!

Following up on the questioner from Ch. 4.

> "For ten years, I've been troubled by my metastasizing cancer. After a reading from Master Okawa, it was revealed that the cause of my cancer was in my past life. Furthermore, for my present life, I was advised to not only value justice but to nurture a heart of compassion. During the reading, I felt a strange sensation that made my affected areas become warm. Then, subsequent medical screenings revealed that the large cancer shadows around my breasts had disappeared and the metastasis had completely stopped. It was a miracle I can never be grateful enough."
>
> (Ms. N.I.)

Testimony 3 — AFTER MY SPACE PEOPLE READING, MY ATOPIC DERMATITIS HEALED!

Case example introduced in Ch. 3.

> "Since I was five, I suffered from the pain and itchiness of atopic dermatitis. However, August 2011 marked a major turning point in my life. I was given an opportunity to have Master Okawa's reading conducted on me, which revealed that in the past, I was actually a space people dwelling underground in Mars. Furthermore, Master Okawa encouraged me saying that he felt within me a power that can even break through tunnels. I was finally able to accept myself for who I truly am, and I was filled with happiness and gratitude. Soon after that, my skin condition improved and it is now healthy and smooth."
>
> (Mr. K.K.)

Testimony 4 — MY 3.5 INCHES (9CM) LARGE, LATE STAGE BREAST CANCER, COMPLETELY CURED!

"A few years ago, I was given a prognosis of having only four months to live due to a late stage breast cancer. After watching Master Okawa's lecture I decided to cure my cancer with the power of thoughts, because I learned that cancer is something created by own mind. So I continued to practice self-reflection, gratitude, spiritual training and prayer. Then the large nine-centimeter (3.5 inches) cancer started to shrink in size. Afterwards, I took a kigan (ritual prayer), 'Prayer to Eradicate Cancer Cells,' and at a subsequent examination, I found that my cancer cells had completely disappeared."

(Ms. K.K.)

Testimony 5 — I BECAME MUCH HEALTHIER AFTER TAKING A RITUAL PRAYER!

Case example of the questionnaire, introduced in Ch. 3.

"In my case, whenever I take 'Prayer for Doubling Your Health' at Hakone Shoja, my blood glucose level drops dramatically, which always surprises me. When I was diagnosed as angina pectoris, it was found that a natural bypass blood vessel developed right next to my clogged blood vessel. The doctor had told me, 'If the bypass had not grown, your chance of death would have been 99%.' I believe this was the blessing of the kigan and I am very grateful."

(Mr. H.)

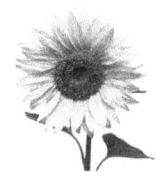

Ritual Prayers for You
to Receive Healing Light from Heaven and Overcome Illness

At Happy Science, we hold many ritual prayers to help you recover from illness and regain health in your life. Here are some of the ritual prayers you can take.

Prayer to Eradicate Cancer Cells

You will ask the Lord to forgive you for having a mind that causes cancer and for the sins committed in your past lives. The Light of the Lord will eradicate the cancer cells in your body.

Prayer for Preventing Infectious Disease

You will pray for protection from all infectious diseases. The prayer states the types of mindset that will keep malignant viruses away from you.

Prayer for Defeating Infectious Disease

In the name of Lord, this prayer will reprimand and defeat the malignant viruses that are plaguing your holy body given to you for soul training.

Preventing Pollen Allergies
—Super Powerful Healing Prayer

You will pray to Ophealis, the great god of mystics, for his protection against all pathological changes and health problems caused by pollen and for a much better health.

Super Vega Healing
—The Miraculous Power of the Goddess Isis—

You will receive a miraculous power of regeneration from Planet Vega, a planet of evolution, progress and transformation. Medical technology on Vega is a thousand years ahead of that on Earth.

Prayer for Doubling Our Health

A miraculous and mystical ritual prayer guided by Ophealis, a god with vast spiritual powers. You will pray to remove all kinds of obstacles in life.

<u>MONTHLY PRAYER CEREMONY</u>
Prayer for Recovery from Illness
Prayer for Health

-Other ritual prayers are also available.
Please contact your nearest temple or branch.

* The main temples at Happy Science are facilities used for religious seminars. They are sacred places where light shines down from Heaven. You may discover your true self full of energy as you get enveloped in warm, gentle light.

The Merits of
The True Words Spoken By Buddha

The main sutra (prayer) of Happy Science is *The True Words Spoken By Buddha*. This prayer contains the fundamental teachings of Happy Science and many books published by Master Ryuho Okawa are extensive explanations of this sutra. Various miracles are being reported from all around the world by reciting this prayer.

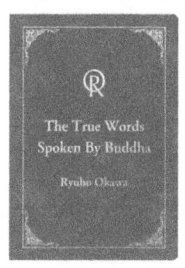

Members can receive this sutra book.

Testimony 6 A MIRACULOUS REVIVAL FROM THE BRINK OF DEATH!

"I was taking care of my wife who was in her late stages of cancer, and one day a friend told me, 'Read this, your wife will surely become better,' and suggested I recite 'The True Words Spoken By Buddha.' On the eighth day of reciting it, my wife who had been complaining that she would rather die than stay alive, suddenly started to regain her appetite. She then started to recover very quickly and after one month, she was able to leave the hospital. The recovery was as if she came back to life. Even the doctor was surprised, claiming that it was a miracle. It was a painful experience of illness, but perhaps this was our chance to encounter faith. Since then, we recite 'The True Words Spoken By Buddha' every single day without fail." (Mr. K. F.)

ABOUT THE AUTHOR

Founder and CEO of Happy Science Group.

Ryuho Okawa was born on July 7th 1956, in Tokushima, Japan. After graduating from the University of Tokyo with a law degree, he joined a Tokyo-based trading house. While working at its New York headquarters, he studied international finance at the Graduate Center of the City University of New York. In 1981, he attained Great Enlightenment and became aware that he is El Cantare with a mission to bring salvation to all humankind.

In 1986, he established Happy Science. It now has members in over 165 countries across the world, with more than 700 branches and temples as well as 10,000 missionary houses around the world.

He has given over 3,450 lectures (of which more than 150 are in English) and published over 3,000 books (of which more than 600 are Spiritual Interview Series), and many are translated into 40 languages. Along with *The Laws of the Sun* and *The Laws Of Messiah*, many of the books have become best sellers or million sellers. To date, Happy Science has produced 25 movies. The original story and original concept were given by the Executive Producer Ryuho Okawa. He has also composed music and written lyrics of over 450 pieces.

Moreover, he is the Founder of Happy Science University and Happy Science Academy (Junior and Senior High School), Founder and President of the Happiness Realization Party, Founder and Honorary Headmaster of Happy Science Institute of Government and Management, Founder of IRH Press Co., Ltd., and the Chairperson of NEW STAR PRODUCTION Co., Ltd. and ARI Production Co., Ltd.

WHAT IS EL CANTARE?

El Cantare means "the Light of the Earth," and is the Supreme God of the Earth who has been guiding humankind since the beginning of Genesis. He is whom Jesus called Father and Muhammad called Allah, and is *Ame-no-Mioya-Gami*, Japanese Father God. Different parts of El Cantare's core consciousness have descended to Earth in the past, once as Alpha and another as Elohim. His branch spirits, such as Shakyamuni Buddha and Hermes, have descended to Earth many times and helped to flourish many civilizations. To unite various religions and to integrate various fields of study in order to build a new civilization on Earth, a part of the core consciousness has descended to Earth as Master Ryuho Okawa.

Alpha is a part of the core consciousness of El Cantare who descended to Earth around 330 million years ago. Alpha preached Earth's Truths to harmonize and unify Earth-born humans and space people who came from other planets.

Elohim is a part of El Cantare's core consciousness who descended to Earth around 150 million years ago. He gave wisdom, mainly on the differences of light and darkness, good and evil.

Ame-no-Mioya-Gami (Japanese Father God) is the Creator God and the Father God who appears in the ancient literature, *Hotsuma Tsutae*. It is believed that He descended on the foothills of Mt. Fuji about 30,000 years ago and built the Fuji dynasty, which is the root of the Japanese civilization. With justice as the central pillar, Ame-no-Mioya-Gami's teachings spread to ancient civilizations of other countries in the world.

Shakyamuni Buddha was born as a prince into the Shakya Clan in India around 2,600 years ago. When he was 29 years old, he renounced the world and sought enlightenment. He later attained Great Enlightenment and founded Buddhism.

Hermes is one of the 12 Olympian gods in Greek mythology, but the spiritual Truth is that he taught the teachings of love and progress around 4,300 years ago that became the origin of the current Western civilization. He is a hero that truly existed.

Ophealis was born in Greece around 6,500 years ago and was the leader who took an expedition to as far as Egypt. He is the God of miracles, prosperity, and arts, and is known as Osiris in the Egyptian mythology.

Rient Arl Croud was born as a king of the ancient Incan Empire around 7,000 years ago and taught about the mysteries of the mind. In the heavenly world, he is responsible for the interactions that take place between various planets.

Thoth was an almighty leader who built the golden age of the Atlantic civilization around 12,000 years ago. In the Egyptian mythology, he is known as god Thoth.

Ra Mu was a leader who built the golden age of the civilization of Mu around 17,000 years ago. As a religious leader and a politician, he ruled by uniting religion and politics.

ABOUT HAPPY SCIENCE

Happy Science is a global movement that empowers individuals to find purpose and spiritual happiness and to share that happiness with their families, societies, and the world. With more than 12 million members around the world, Happy Science aims to increase awareness of spiritual truths and expand our capacity for love, compassion, and joy so that together we can create the kind of world we all wish to live in.

Activities at Happy Science are based on the Principle of Happiness (Love, Wisdom, Self-Reflection, and Progress). This principle embraces worldwide philosophies and beliefs, transcending boundaries of culture and religions.

> **Love** teaches us to give ourselves freely without expecting anything in return; it encompasses giving, nurturing, and forgiving.
>
> **Wisdom** leads us to the insights of spiritual truths, and opens us to the true meaning of life and the will of God (the universe, the highest power, Buddha).
>
> **Self-Reflection** brings a mindful, nonjudgmental lens to our thoughts and actions to help us find our truest selves—the essence of our souls—and deepen our connection to the highest power. It helps us attain a clean and peaceful mind and leads us to the right life path.

Progress emphasizes the positive, dynamic aspects of our spiritual growth—actions we can take to manifest and spread happiness around the world. It's a path that not only expands our soul growth, but also furthers the collective potential of the world we live in.

PROGRAMS AND EVENTS

The doors of Happy Science are open to all. We offer a variety of programs and events, including self-exploration and self-growth programs, spiritual seminars, meditation and contemplation sessions, study groups, and book events.

Our programs are designed to:
* Deepen your understanding of your purpose and meaning in life
* Improve your relationships and increase your capacity to love unconditionally
* Attain peace of mind, decrease anxiety and stress, and feel positive
* Gain deeper insights and a broader perspective on the world
* Learn how to overcome life's challenges
  ... and much more.

For more information, visit happy-science.org.

OUR ACTIVITIES

Happy Science does other various activities to provide support for those in need.

- **You Are An Angel! General Incorporated Association**
Happy Science has a volunteer network in Japan that encourages and supports children with disabilities as well as their parents and guardians.

- **Never Mind School for Truancy**
At 'Never Mind,' we support students who find it very challenging to attend schools in Japan. We also nurture their self-help spirit and power to rebound against obstacles in life based on Master Okawa's teachings and faith.

- **"Prevention Against Suicide" Campaign since 2003**
A nationwide campaign to reduce suicides; over 20,000 people commit suicide every year in Japan. "The Suicide Prevention Website-Words of Truth for You-" presents spiritual prescriptions for worries such as depression, lost love, extramarital affairs, bullying and work-related problems, thereby saving many lives.

- **Support for Anti-bullying Campaigns**
Happy Science provides support for a group of parents and guardians, Network to Protect Children from Bullying, a general incorporated foundation launched in Japan to end bullying, including those that can even be called a criminal offense. So far, the network received more than 5,000 cases and resolved 90% of them.

- **The Golden Age Scholarship**
  This scholarship is granted to students who can contribute greatly and bring a hopeful future to the world.

- **Success No.1**
  Buddha's Truth Afterschool Academy
  Happy Science has over 180 classrooms throughout Japan and in several cities around the world that focus on afterschool education for children. The education focuses on faith and morals in addition to supporting children's school studies.

- **Angel Plan V**
  For children under the age of kindergarten, Happy Science holds classes for nurturing healthy, positive, and creative boys and girls.

- **Future Stars Training Department**
  The Future Stars Training Department was founded within the Happy Science Media Division with the goal of nurturing talented individuals to become successful in the performing arts and entertainment industry.

- **NEW STAR PRODUCTION Co., Ltd.**
  ARI Production Co., Ltd.
  We have companies to nurture actors and actresses, artists, and vocalists. They are also involved in film production.

CONTACT INFORMATION

Happy Science is a worldwide organization with branches and temples around the globe. For a comprehensive list, visit the worldwide directory at *happy-science.org*. The following are some of the many Happy Science locations:

UNITED STATES AND CANADA

New York
79 Franklin St., New York, NY 10013, USA
Phone: 1-212-343-7972
Fax: 1-212-343-7973
Email: ny@happy-science.org
Website: happyscience-usa.org

New Jersey
66 Hudson St., #2R, Hoboken, NJ 07030, USA
Phone: 1-201-313-0127
Email: nj@happy-science.org
Website: happyscience-usa.org

Chicago
2300 Barrington Rd., Suite #400,
Hoffman Estates, IL 60169, USA
Phone: 1-630-937-3077
Email: chicago@happy-science.org
Website: happyscience-usa.org

Florida
5208 8th St., Zephyrhills, FL 33542, USA
Phone: 1-813-715-0000
Fax: 1-813-715-0010
Email: florida@happy-science.org
Website: happyscience-usa.org

Atlanta
1874 Piedmont Ave., NE Suite 360-C
Atlanta, GA 30324, USA
Phone: 1-404-892-7770
Email: atlanta@happy-science.org
Website: happyscience-usa.org

San Francisco
525 Clinton St.
Redwood City, CA 94062, USA
Phone & Fax: 1-650-363-2777
Email: sf@happy-science.org
Website: happyscience-usa.org

Los Angeles
1590 E. Del Mar Blvd., Pasadena, CA 91106, USA
Phone: 1-626-395-7775
Fax: 1-626-395-7776
Email: la@happy-science.org
Website: happyscience-usa.org

Orange County
16541 Gothard St. Suite 104
Huntington Beach, CA 92647
Phone: 1-714-659-1501
Email: oc@happy-science.org
Website: happyscience-usa.org

San Diego
7841 Balboa Ave. Suite #202
San Diego, CA 92111, USA
Phone: 1-626-395-7775
Fax: 1-626-395-7776
E-mail: sandiego@happy-science.org
Website: happyscience-usa.org

Hawaii
Phone: 1-808-591-9772
Fax: 1-808-591-9776
Email: hi@happy-science.org
Website: happyscience-usa.org

Kauai
3343 Kanakolu Street, Suite 5
Lihue, HI 96766, USA
Phone: 1-808-822-7007
Fax: 1-808-822-6007
Email: kauai-hi@happy-science.org
Website: happyscience-usa.org

Toronto
845 The Queensway
Etobicoke, ON M8Z 1N6, Canada
Phone: 1-416-901-3747
Email: toronto@happy-science.org
Website: happy-science.ca

Vancouver
#201-2607 East 49th Avenue,
Vancouver, BC, V5S 1J9, Canada
Phone: 1-604-437-7735
Fax: 1-604-437-7764
Email: vancouver@happy-science.org
Website: happy-science.ca

INTERNATIONAL

Tokyo
1-6-7 Togoshi, Shinagawa,
Tokyo, 142-0041, Japan
Phone: 81-3-6384-5770
Fax: 81-3-6384-5776
Email: tokyo@happy-science.org
Website: happy-science.org

Seoul
74, Sadang-ro 27-gil,
Dongjak-gu, Seoul, Korea
Phone: 82-2-3478-8777
Fax: 82-2-3478-9777
Email: korea@happy-science.org
Website: happyscience-korea.org

London
3 Margaret St.
London, W1W 8RE United Kingdom
Phone: 44-20-7323-9255
Fax: 44-20-7323-9344
Email: eu@happy-science.org
Website: www.happyscience-uk.org

Taipei
No. 89, Lane 155, Dunhua N. Road,
Songshan District, Taipei City 105, Taiwan
Phone: 886-2-2719-9377
Fax: 886-2-2719-5570
Email: taiwan@happy-science.org
Website: happyscience-tw.org

Sydney
516 Pacific Highway, Lane Cove North,
2066 NSW, Australia
Phone: 61-2-9411-2877
Fax: 61-2-9411-2822
Email: sydney@happy-science.org

Kuala Lumpur
No 22A, Block 2, Jalil Link Jalan Jalil
Jaya 2, Bukit Jalil 57000,
Kuala Lumpur, Malaysia
Phone: 60-3-8998-7877
Fax: 60-3-8998-7977
Email: malaysia@happy-science.org
Website: happyscience.org.my

Sao Paulo
Rua. Domingos de Morais 1154,
Vila Mariana, Sao Paulo SP
CEP 04010-100, Brazil
Phone: 55-11-5088-3800
Email: sp@happy-science.org
Website: happyscience.com.br

Kathmandu
Kathmandu Metropolitan City,
Ward No. 15, Ring Road, Kimdol,
Sitapaila Kathmandu, Nepal
Phone: 977-1-427-2931
Email: nepal@happy-science.org

Jundiai
Rua Congo, 447, Jd. Bonfiglioli
Jundiai-CEP, 13207-340, Brazil
Phone: 55-11-4587-5952
Email: jundiai@happy-science.org

Kampala
Plot 877 Rubaga Road, Kampala
P.O. Box 34130 Kampala, UGANDA
Phone: 256-79-4682-121
Email: uganda@happy-science.org

ABOUT HAPPINESS REALIZATION PARTY

The Happiness Realization Party (HRP) was founded in May 2009 by Master Ryuho Okawa as part of the Happy Science Group. HRP strives to improve the Japanese society, based on three basic political principles of "freedom, democracy, and faith," and let Japan promote individual and public happiness from Asia to the world as a leader nation.

1) Diplomacy and Security: Protecting Freedom, Democracy, and Faith of Japan and the World from China's Totalitarianism

Japan's current defense system is insufficient against China's expanding hegemony and the threat of North Korea's nuclear missiles. Japan, as the leader of Asia, must strengthen its defense power and promote strategic diplomacy together with the nations which share the values of freedom, democracy, and faith. Further, HRP aims to realize world peace under the leadership of Japan, the nation with the spirit of religious tolerance.

2) Economy: Early economic recovery through utilizing the "wisdom of the private sector"

Economy has been damaged severely by the novel coronavirus originated in China. Many companies have been forced into bankruptcy or out of business. What is needed for economic recovery now is not subsidies and regulations by the government, but policies which can utilize the "wisdom of the private sector."

For more information, visit en.hr-party.jp

HAPPY SCIENCE ACADEMY JUNIOR AND SENIOR HIGH SCHOOL

Happy Science Academy Junior and Senior High School is a boarding school founded with the goal of educating the future leaders of the world who can have a big vision, persevere, and take on new challenges.

Currently, there are two campuses in Japan; the Nasu Main Campus in Tochigi Prefecture, founded in 2010, and the Kansai Campus in Shiga Prefecture, founded in 2013.

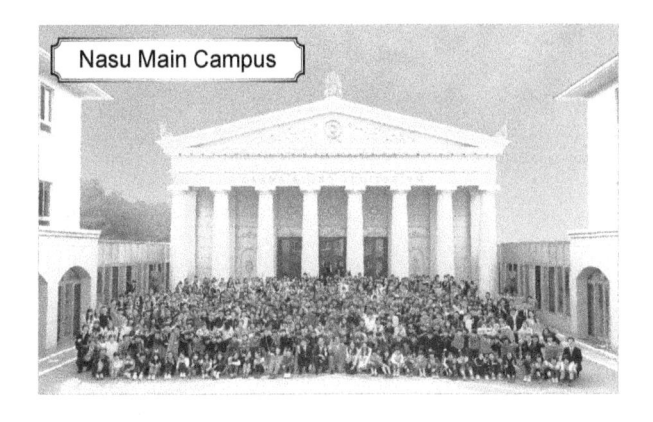

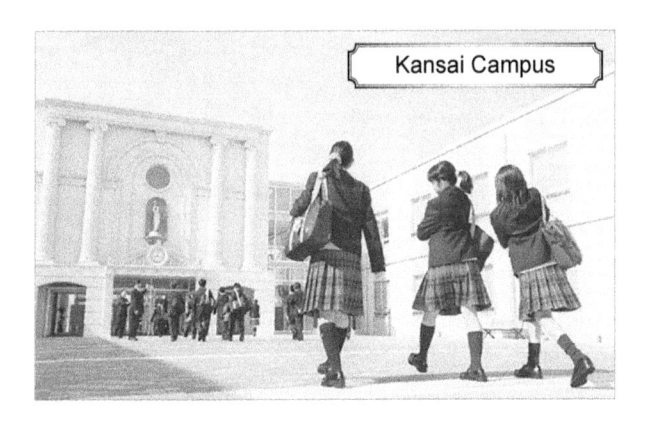

Nasu Main Campus

Kansai Campus

HAPPY SCIENCE UNIVERSITY

THE FOUNDING SPIRIT AND THE GOAL OF EDUCATION

Based on the founding philosophy of the university, "Exploration of happiness and the creation of a new civilization," education, research and studies will be provided to help students acquire deep understanding grounded in religious belief and advanced expertise with the objectives of producing "great talents of virtue" who can contribute in a broad-ranging way to serve Japan and the international society.

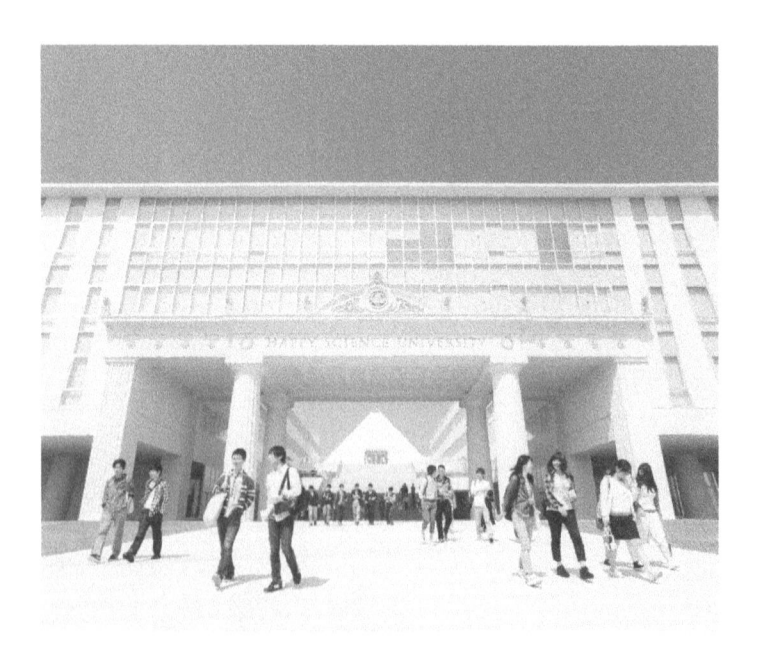

FACULTIES

Faculty of human happiness

Students in this faculty will pursue liberal arts from various perspectives with a multidisciplinary approach, explore and envision an ideal state of human beings and society.

Faculty of successful management

This faculty aims to realize successful management that helps organizations to create value and wealth for society and to contribute to the happiness and the development of management and employees as well as society as a whole.

Faculty of future creation

Students in this faculty study subjects such as political science, journalism, performing arts and artistic expression, and explore and present new political and cultural models based on truth, goodness and beauty.

Faculty of future industry

This faculty aims to nurture engineers who can resolve various issues facing modern civilization from a technological standpoint and contribute to the creation of new industries of the future.

ABOUT HS PRESS

HS Press is an imprint of IRH Press Co., Ltd. IRH Press Co., Ltd., based in Tokyo, was founded in 1987 as a publishing division of Happy Science. IRH Press publishes religious and spiritual books, journals, magazines and also operates broadcast and film production enterprises. For more information, visit *okawabooks.com*.

Follow us on:

- Facebook: Okawa Books
- Youtube: Okawa Books
- Pinterest: Okawa Books
- Instagram: OkawaBooks
- Twitter: Okawa Books
- Goodreads: Ryuho Okawa

NEWSLETTER

To receive book related news, promotions and events, please subscribe to our newsletter below.

eepurl.com/bsMeJj

AUDIO / VISUAL MEDIA

YOUTUBE

PODCAST

Introduction of Ryuho Okawa's titles; topics ranging from self-help, current affairs, spirituality, religion, and the universe.

BOOKS BY RYUHO OKAWA

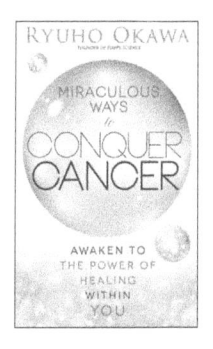

MIRACULOUS WAYS TO CONQUER CANCER
Awaken to the Power of Healing within You

Why do people get cancer? Why does the number of patients with cancer keep increasing in spite of medical progress? This book reveals how the mind creates cancer and the keys to overcome illnesses. Drive out cancer from your life!

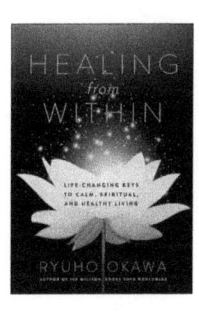

Healing from Within
Life-Changing Keys to Calm, Spiritual, and Healthy Living

The true causes and remedies for various illnesses that modern medicine doesn't know how to cure are revealed in this book. By following the steps that are suggested here, you will gain new perspective on the relationship between mind and body.

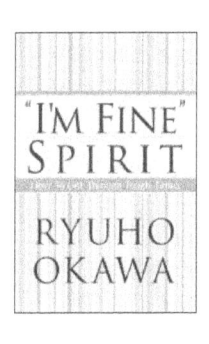

"I'M FINE" SPIRIT

This book is filled with wisdom that you can use to help you bring back your smile and restore your health. You will be bright and clear as a sunny day. Let's turn your worries into seeds of happiness.

[This book is available only in local branches and temples. Please refer to the contact information.]

For a complete list of books, visit okawabooks.com

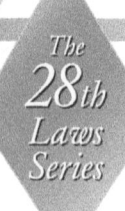

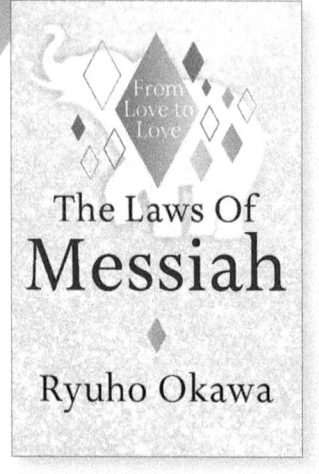

The Laws Of Messiah
From Love to Love

Paperback • 248 pages • $16.95
ISBN: 978-1-942125-90-7 (Jan. 31, 2022)

"What is Messiah?" This book carries an important message of love and guidance to people living now from the Modern-Day Messiah or the Modern-Day Savior. It also reveals the secret of Shambhala, the spiritual center of Earth, as well as the truth that this spiritual center is currently in danger of perishing and what we can do to protect this sacred place.

Love your Lord God. Know that those who don't know love don't know God. Discover the true love of God and the ideal practice of faith. This book teaches the most important element we must not lose sight of as we go through our soul training on this planet Earth.

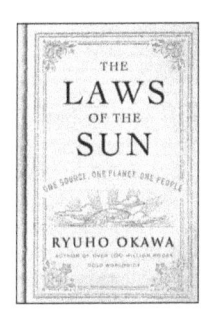

THE LAWS OF THE SUN
ONE SOURCE, ONE PLANET, ONE PEOPLE

IMAGINE IF YOU COULD ASK GOD why He created this world and what spiritual laws He used to shape us—and everything around us. If we could understand His designs and intentions, we could discover what our goals in life should be and whether our actions move us closer to those goals or farther away.

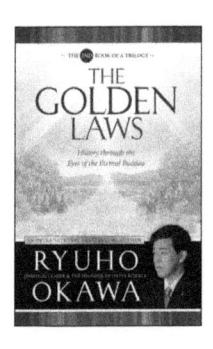

THE GOLDEN LAWS
HISTORY THROUGH THE EYES OF THE ETERNAL BUDDHA

The Golden Laws reveals how Buddha's Plan has been unfolding on earth, and outlines five thousand years of the secret history of humankind. Once we understand the true course of history, we cannot help but become aware of the significance of our spiritual mission in the present age.

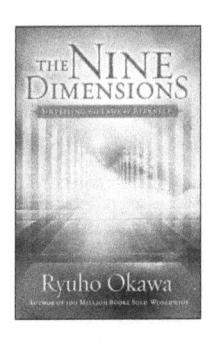

THE NINE DIMENSIONS
UNVEILING THE LAWS OF ETERNITY

This book is a window into the mind of our loving God, who encourages us to grow into greater angels. It reveals His deepest intentions, answering the timely question of why He conceived such a colorful medley of religions, philosophies, sciences, arts, and other forms of expression.

For a complete list of books, visit okawabooks.com

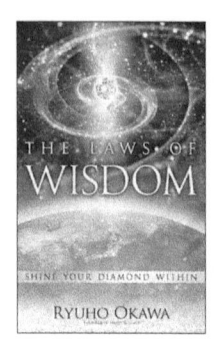

THE LAWS OF WISDOM
SHINE YOUR DIAMOND WITHIN

This book guides you along the path on how to acquire wisdom, so that you can break through any wall you are facing or will confront in your life or in your business. By reading this book, you will be able to avoid getting lost in the flood of information and go beyond the level of just amassing knowledge. You will be able to come up with many great ideas, make effective planning and strategy and develop your leadership while receiving good inspiration.

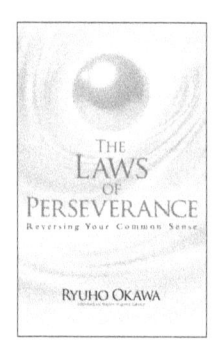

THE LAWS OF PERSEVERANCE
REVERSING YOUR COMMON SENSE

"No matter how much you suffer, the Truth will gradually shine forth as you continue to endure hardships. Therefore, simply strengthen your mind and keep making constant efforts in times of endurance, however ordinary they may be."

-From Postscript

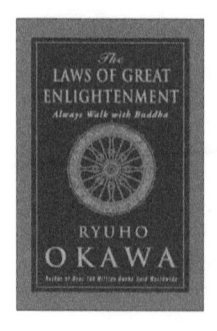

THE LAWS OF GREAT ENLIGHTENMENT
ALWAYS WALK WITH BUDDHA

In this modern society, we often find ourselves unable to forgive someone and maintain a peaceful mind. However, there are ways to lead a stress-free life and enjoy happiness from within. This book offers the practical approaches to achieve it. By understanding the Buddhist concept "enlightenment," you will gain the power to forgive sins and get to know how to be the master of your own mind.

For a complete list of books, visit okawabooks.com

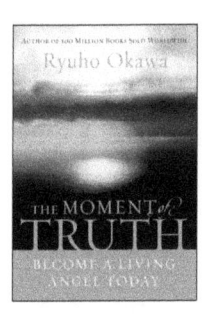

THE MOMENT OF TRUTH

BECOME A LIVING ANGEL TODAY

This book shows that we are essentially spiritual beings and that our true and lasting happiness is not found within the material world but rather in acts of unconditional and selfless love toward the greater world. These pages reveal God's mind, His mercy, and His hope that many of us will become living angels that shine light onto this world.

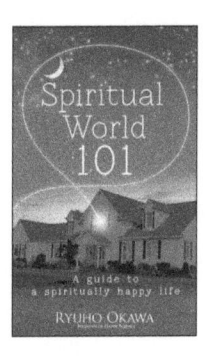

SPIRITUAL WORLD 101

A GUIDE TO A SPIRITUALLY HAPPY LIFE

This book is a spiritual guidebook that will answer all your questions about the spiritual world, with illustrations and diagrams explaining about your guardian spirit and the secrets of God and Buddha. By reading this book, you will be able to understand the true meaning of life and find happiness in everyday life.

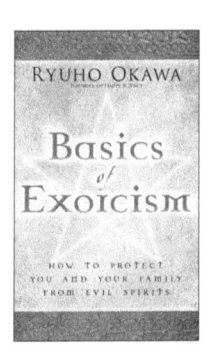

BASICS OF EXORCISM

HOW TO PROTECT YOU AND YOUR FAMILY FROM EVIL SPIRITS

No matter how much time progresses, demons are real. Spiritual screen against curses - the truth of exorcism as told by the author who possesses the six great supernatural powers - The essence of exorcism as a result of more than 5000 rounds of exorcist experience!

For a complete list of books, visit okawabooks.com

Ingram Content Group UK Ltd.
Milton Keynes UK
UKHW011816190323
418793UK00001B/319